Pr

THE WELLNESS

"Reena has given us a book filled with wisdom about health and wellness, but the learnings and insights extend far beyond that. They touch our heart, mind, spirit, and body! Reena shares how to live a Passion Fit life, a life that is consistently aligning wellness to one's values and personal mission. In addition to giving readers an inspiring book, she also gives us a practical one. Each chapter ends with self-reflection questions to support the reader's journey to truly living a wellness-evolved life."

—**Camille van den Broeck**, Founder of Camille's Leadership and Coaching Services, and Former Sales and Go-to-Market Business Partner at Google

"I'm truly honored to call Reena a friend and colleague! She has contributed to our Emmy-nominated lifestyle and entertainment show by bringing her incredible knowledge, when it comes to health and wellness, to the table. This book has so much to offer women who want practical advice to improve their lives!"

—**Ashley Jacobs**, TV Host of Fox 5 San Diego's The LOCAList SD

"*The Wellness-Evolved Woman* inspired me to look into my own journey of self-love and self-care. It offers practical tips for women to build a stronger connection with themselves. In the last year, I have learned to accept change through a new job, and Reena's next book encouraged me to think about my past, present challenges, and future goals. The Wellness-Evolved Woman teaches us to find significance in our life experiences, helping us discover our unique purposes."

—**Kathleen Ferguson**, Founder and CEO of Coach360

"*The Wellness-Evolved Woman* is like having a trusted friend by your side, guiding you through the ups and downs of life with wisdom and grace. This book is a true gift for any woman ready to grow and thrive."

—**Kelsey Johnston**, Marketing Consultant at Fox 5 San Diego and Adjunct Professor of Media and Communications at University of San Diego

THE
WELLNESS-EVOLVED WOMAN

EMBRACING YOUR AUTHENTIC SELF THROUGHOUT YOUR PASSION FIT LIFE

REENA VOKOUN

FUCHSIA ROSE
MEDIA

**The Wellness-Evolved Woman: Embracing Your Authentic
Self throughout Your Passion Fit Life**
Published by Fuchsia Rose Media™
San Diego, CA

Names: Vokoun, Reena, author.
Title:The wellness-evolved woman : embracing your authentic self throughout
your Passion Fit life / Reena Vokoun.
Description: San Diego, CA : Fuchsia Rose Media, [2025] | Series: The women's
wellness series. | Includes bibliographical references.
Identifiers: ISBN: 978-1-7363647-1-0
Subjects: LCSH: Self-actualization (Psychology) | Self-realization. | Change
(Psychology) | Mind and body. | Self-care, Health. | Mental health. | Success. |
Achievement motivation in women. | Feminist spirituality. | BISAC: SELF-HELP
/ Personal Growth / Success. | SELF-HELP / Personal Growth / Happiness.
Classification: LCC: BF637.S4 V65 2025 | DDC: 158.1–dc23

Cover and Interior Design by Victoria Wolf, wolfdesignandmarketing.com
Book Cover Photography by Marcy Browe Photography
Author Bio Photography by Jessica Faehnle at Napier J Photography

QUANTITY PURCHASES: Schools, companies, professional groups, clubs, and
other organizations may qualify for special terms when ordering quantities of this
title. For information, email contact@fuchsiarosemedia.com.

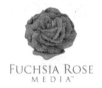

FUCHSIA ROSE
M E D I A™

To my immediate and extended family members, who have all played a prominent role in shaping me into the woman I am today—this book is for you, as a token of my love and appreciation for being my core family, my foundation, my home.

CONTENTS

A DEEPER LOOK
INTO MY STORY

WHEN I WAS NINETEEN YEARS OLD and a sophomore in college, I took Stephen Covey's The 7 Habits of Highly Effective People Leadership Course within the business school and was inspired at that time by both the course and Covey's book. One of the topics we discussed was identifying our values and writing out our personal vision and a mission statement for our life.

I knew I wanted to write my mission statement in such a way that I could read it decades later, hoping that my deepest values, goals, and aspirations would still hold true—and that I'd be able to live them out over the course of my lifetime. All these years later, I can honestly say that everything I wrote then is still true to the core of me, even though I've also grown and evolved since then.

I've experienced and accomplished many of the goals I set for myself, and I've had incredible support through the years in doing so. I'm grateful for my loving and supportive family of origin, including my sweet grandparents, parents, two brothers, and sister. I'm grateful for my higher education and career, including having had the opportunity to work for some extremely innovative companies that have had a positive impact in the world before founding and launching my own company, Passion Fit, where I'm able to do my life's work in the health and wellness industry. I'm grateful that after growing up in the Midwest and living on the East and West Coasts, I'm able to call my dream state of California home. I'm grateful to have met my amazing husband a few years after college, and I'm grateful for the loving and supportive family he and I have created with our two incredible sons, who are the greatest gifts we could have ever asked for in life. I'm also grateful for my wonderful extended family and in-laws, as well as the deep, treasured, and lifelong friendships I've made through various stages of my life.

Throughout my journey so far, I've also gone through difficult times, experienced self-doubt, faced fears, felt lost, and didn't feel I was living up to my full potential. I share more in-depth thoughts about my personal story throughout *The Wellness-Evolved Woman.* What I've come to understand and appreciate is that through the ups and downs of life, my mission statement has been a constant, like a guiding star, always pointing me back to my authentic self and the way

I want to live my life and serve others. I had no idea when I wrote it all those years ago that it would lead me to understand what it means to be a wellness-evolved woman.

When I first set out to write this wellness book series for women over ten years ago, and before even launching my company, my goal was for these books to be relevant, timeless, nonjudgmental, insightful, motivating, and inspiring for women of all ages, and backgrounds. I also wanted this series to include both a depth and breadth of ideas, information, and perspectives on physical, mental, emotional, and spiritual health, as well as personal and professional development, to make it applicable to women, both despite and in spite of the different life stages they might be in. The series could also serve as a way for women to learn from their past, understand their present, and prepare for their future, much like I set out to do when I wrote my mission statement many years ago.

In my first book, *The Wellness-Empowered Woman*, I focused on female empowerment, professional development, and health and wellness, covering topics such as mindfulness, stress, anxiety, sleep, exercise, nutrition, work-life balance, perfectionism, failure, and community. I wrote about these topics because I'd experienced my own struggles in the past, trying to balance my career with my family while dealing with burnout, health issues, and a sense of failure. I knew other women might be experiencing the same challenges, so I wanted to take my experiences, learnings, and trainings and help women succeed both personally and professionally through wellness.

In this follow-up book, I go deeper into your mental and emotional health and the impacts they can have on your physical health, relationships, career, and more, especially as you continue to evolve throughout your life. Diving deeper into your mental and emotional health can often cause a myriad of emotions to surface, which it certainly has for me. I am personally experiencing the importance of going deeper, as I am now a mom of teen boys, I have been married to my husband for over twenty years, and I am in my tenth year of being an entrepreneur and running my company. I've come to realize that being a wellness-evolved woman means I'm willing to learn and grow through each phase and stage of life.

The Wellness-Empowered Woman focused on self-care, which is essential when we begin to discover the importance of prioritizing our own well-being. In this book, I shine a light on the need for us to evolve beyond that place of self-care into a deeper place of self-love, which can help us embrace the inevitable changes that happen in life. Being rooted in self-love and having ongoing wellness tools to help us through evolution and change are key to finding true and lasting happiness; experiencing unconditional love for ourselves, our families, and our friends; and enjoying peace, good health, and personal and professional success during our lifetime.

Throughout this book, I offer insights on growing from a wellness-empowered woman to a wellness-evolved woman, what it means to live a Passion Fit life through different life stages, and the relationship between self-love and self-care. You will also have the opportunity to reflect on where you've been, where you are, and where you're going, embracing change throughout, since it's our only constant in life. We will also look at how ethnicity and authenticity go hand in hand.

I'll share why leveraging your innate talents, strengths, and skills can be a blueprint for success, and how your interests can connect you to others. In addition, I'll cover how to find meaning in your life experiences, how education can be your foundation, and how your core values can guide you through the journey of life.

Finally, I'll reveal and reflect on my personal mission statement decades after I wrote it, and you'll have the opportunity to discover your own mission in life, if you haven't already. Throughout the book, along with stories from my life, I'll share learnings from public figures and anonymous examples from my work with clients as well.

And just as I did in my first book, I invite you to grab a notebook. Or feel free to get your own *The Wellness-Empowered Woman* or *The Wellness-Evolved Woman* notebooks, which are available on the Passion Fit online boutique! I encourage you to write out your answers to the reflection questions at the end of each chapter. Going through this process will allow you to get the most out of this book, and you will have your thoughts, ideas, and reflections as reference points for the future.

Get ready for a life-changing adventure, as you take becoming a wellness-empowered woman to the next level and become a wellness-evolved woman. Please know you have all my love and support, and I'll continue to guide you as a trusted friend on this wellness journey of a lifetime!

CHAPTER 1

GOING FROM A WELLNESS-EMPOWERED WOMAN TO A WELLNESS-EVOLVED WOMAN

AS WE BEGIN OUR JOURNEY TOGETHER in *The Wellness-Evolved Woman*, it is essential that we uncover what it means to go from being a wellness-empowered woman to becoming a wellness-evolved woman. In the simplest of terms, it means taking all the knowledge, skills, and tools you have learned to become empowered through wellness and applying them to your life on an ongoing basis, both in good times and challenging times, as you evolve and grow as a person over time.

For example, I was a wellness-empowered woman throughout my teenage and young adult years. Despite high school, college, work, marriage, graduate school, and other responsibilities, I prioritized my workouts, healthy eating, management of stress through mindfulness and deep breathing, and my need for plenty of sleep. But once my career became more demanding and my husband and I had kids, I lost sight of that empowerment for several years. This led to my burnout and health issues.

While I'm grateful I was able to find my way back to wellness, especially since it's always been such a huge passion of mine, I wanted to make sure those wellness practices, tools, and values became so heavily ingrained into my habits and life that no matter what stages or circumstances arose, I would be able to maintain that empowerment—or continue to come back to it—over and over again. To me, that's the true essence of progressing from being empowered to being evolved through wellness.

So how do you achieve that? Read on to find out!

As women, we will go through many stages of life that will affect us physically, mentally, emotionally, and maybe even spiritually. From puberty to pregnancy to postpartum to perimenopause to menopause and beyond, our bodies and hormones will inevitably change. While that can be a daunting thought at times, it's part of our evolution from being a little girl to a teenager to a young woman to a middle-aged woman to a woman in her golden years. We may also go through various levels of change through our schooling, jobs, careers, and business endeavors; dating, marriage, and relationship changes; having pets and kids; experiencing health issues; caring for elderly parents; losing loved ones; and more. All of these changes and stages can bring about a tremendous amount of successes, failures, learnings, growth, and wisdom, as well as stress, anxiety, fear, faith, courage, and victory.

Having established wellness practices, tools, and values in place throughout our lives can help us not only survive but thrive. Consistently sleeping well, eating well, moving well, breathing well, and communicating well on an ongoing basis can do wonders for our overall health and well-being and will allow us to cross that bridge from being wellness-empowered to wellness-evolved.

One of my clients who had worked hard to become empowered to establish her wellness practices had gone from working part time while her kids were younger to going back to work full time when they got older. Her family was also building and moving into a new house at that time. She clearly had a lot going on in her life, and we talked about it in our wellness coaching sessions. Since she was stressed due to the change in her work environment and workload, along with her never-ending personal to-do list because of her family's move, it would have been easy for her to let her wellness practices go out the window during that time of transition. However, she tried her best to stay on track with her fitness regimen, nutrition, sleep, and balancing her family and household needs, along with her new full-time job. We worked on creating priorities for her, developing specific and actionable goals, and tackling them one by one. She had times when she was consistent and times when she fell off track a bit, but I reassured her it was all part of the process of evolving and growing. She kept going and is still keeping up with her goals, which is wonderful to see.

Another client worked with me to develop behavior changes to become empowered through nutrition. After several months, she struggled to eat healthy due to her new, demanding corporate job, which required extensive amounts of travel as well. We outlined ways for her to stick to her nutrition plan, being mindful of what she was ordering when she ate out while traveling, as well as how she could meal prep in advance when she was home and prepare healthy meals in thirty minutes or less. It was certainly challenging for her at first, especially when she was tired and jet lagged. We focused on how much more energetic she felt when she ate well and how sluggish she felt when she didn't. We also outlined her original "why" for optimizing her nutrition, eating habits, and health, so she could stay aware of it as her job evolved and changed. She still looks at her "why" often to stay motivated. And, of course, she occasionally indulges, in moderation, in order to enjoy the amazing cuisines in the many cities and countries she visits on her business travels.

It's always a joy to witness my clients prioritizing and re-prioritizing their wellness, even if they step away for a while and come back later. It's an honor to be a constant resource for them. The positive impact I've seen on their health and wellness as a result of their efforts is what drives me to keep working with clients year after year, helping them stay healthy, even as their lives evolve and change. These dedicated women are great examples of going from wellness-empowered to wellness-evolved women.

Two public figures who are also great examples of wellness-evolved women are Denise Austin and Jennifer Aniston.

They both have done an incredible job of consistently managing their busy and impactful careers, personal lives, and health and well-being over many decades. Let's take a look at what makes each of them such great role models.

Denise Austin is a fitness icon and is sixty-seven years old as of the writing of this book. I grew up doing her workout videos on ESPN, which is honestly how I developed a love for fitness at a young age. She's been married to her husband and sports agent, Jeff Austin, for forty years and has been in the fitness industry for that long as well. Together they have two adult daughters, Katie and Kelly Austin, who both have careers in the wellness industry as well.

Throughout her life, Denise Austin has focused on not only helping others stay fit and healthy, but doing so herself and leading by example. Through working out consistently for thirty minutes a day by doing cardio and using light hand weights, walking daily, eating healthy meals without dieting, and focusing on having a positive mindset, she's been able to continue to flourish personally and professionally through each decade of her career and life. She also exudes amazing energy, confidence, and inner and outer beauty. Her longevity, both in her career and healthy lifestyle, is remarkable. Not only has she demonstrated what it means to be an empowered woman, but over the course of her life, she has shown us how to evolve through wellness, honoring each stage along the way.

Jennifer Aniston is a world-famous actress and is fifty-four years old as of this writing. She's most notably known for her roles in TV shows and series, such as *Friends* and *The Morning*

Show, and movies such as *Along Came Polly* and *Rumor Has It*. She was previously married to Brad Pitt and Justin Theroux and is the daughter of late actor, John Aniston, and actress, Nancy Dow. Aniston is heavily involved in philanthropic work for St. Jude Children's Hospital and is a brand partner for Aveeno and Pvolve Fitness. In conjunction with her busy and long-standing career, she's also known for her consistent workouts five to six days per week, including yoga, cardio, and Pilates. She's a big believer in hydration, sleep (after overcoming insomnia), meditation, therapy (which helped her overcome anxiety), self-care, and eating nutritious and balanced meals. Her commitment to a healthy lifestyle is apparent, as she exudes grace, humility, and consistency. She's often referred to in the media as a role model for physical and mental health and well-being.

Through the many personal and professional changes, developments, challenges, and victories during her life, Jennifer Anniston has put her well-being at the center of it all. To me, she's another strong example of what it means to go from empowerment to evolving through wellness during one's life.

As these two incredible women have inspired me to live as a wellness-evolved woman, my hope is that you are inspired by them as well. Here are some tips to maintain your wellness practices as you evolve throughout your life.

Start with your mindset: One of the most important actions you can take for yourself is to have the right mindset. Be clear in your mind that wellness is at the heart of all you will do in your life, both personally and professionally. In order to progress through various stages successfully, it's critical to be able to care for your physical, mental, emotional, and spiritual health. Without these elements of well-being, it's difficult to learn, develop, grow, refine, and renew to your fullest potential. Find ways to remind yourself continuously of these concepts. You might write in a journal, put up reminders at your desk, in your bedroom or bathroom, or make it a part of your daily mindfulness practice. Get creative and figure out the best ways for you to keep your mindset strong and focused on positive health and well-being.

Make wellness a nonnegotiable, daily priority: We all have busy lives, and oftentimes, we have competing priorities. Work is usually a big culprit in not giving ourselves enough time to focus on well-being. In fact, according to Jen Fisher, Paul H. Silverglate, Colleen Bordeaux, and Michael Gilmartin, in an article featured in *Deloitte Insights*, less than two-thirds of employees say their physical and mental well-being are excellent or good.[1] This is becoming an increasing problem both inside and outside the workplace.

If we constantly put our wellness last due to other priorities, it will ultimately catch up with us, and we will suffer in the long term. It's imperative to make wellness a nonnegotiable priority every day. Aim to incorporate at least one or as many wellness practices as possible each day and over the course of each week. For example, prioritize your workouts at least three to five days per week, take some deep breaths every day, cook healthy meals at home at least four to five days per week, and get at least seven hours of sleep every night. By doing so, you're prioritizing some, most, or all of your wellness practices on a daily and weekly basis, which will have a positive impact on your overall health throughout your life.

Create a backup plan when life causes a shift in direction: Life will inevitably throw us some curveballs, and therefore, it's important to have a backup plan, including one for our wellness practices. For example, if a last-minute work trip comes up, try to keep up with your workouts using on-demand videos, mobile apps, or the hotel gym if you won't be able to attend your normal fitness practices that week. Or if you need to attend a work or family dinner instead of cooking at home, order a healthy menu item such as a salad, steamed vegetables, grilled proteins, or a vegan or vegetarian dish to fit into your regular nutrition plan. And if your sleep is negatively impacted by daylight savings time, a late night out on the weekend, or jet lag from travel, use a sleep meditation app, go to bed a little earlier, or invest in some darkening shades or an eye mask to help improve your sleep.

These are just a few examples and ideas for the many scenarios that might pop up in life. The key is to stay as consistent as possible with your wellness practices, even in ever-changing situations. Value yourself and your well-being, and allow your life and wellness practices to be fluid so that you can maintain them to the best of your ability!

Adapt a something-is-better-than-nothing instead of an all-or-nothing mentality: When I work with clients, I often remind them that something is better than nothing when it comes to their health and wellness regimen. Many people take an all-or-nothing approach, which can make it difficult to stay consistent, especially because day-to-day life can be unpredictable. Moving your body for even ten minutes a day, or taking five deep breaths a day, or eating one piece of fruit and one vegetable a day can make a positive difference in your overall health.

Taking this approach can also help to keep wellness in your life for the *rest of your life*, which again, is what being a wellness-evolved woman is all about. So, do what you can, and don't quit if you fall off track or can't commit as much time and energy to your health and wellness regimen as you would like. Every day is a new opportunity to keep going full speed ahead, take baby steps forward, or begin again.

Remember how you feel when wellness is integrated into your life: One of the biggest motivators to integrate wellness into your life consistently is to take note of how it makes you feel. I often ask my clients to take note of how they feel before and after a workout, a healthy meal, a meditation or journaling session, a good night's sleep, a break from work, or time spent with a community. Almost always, clients identify a notable difference.

For instance, I have a client who experiences tightness and pain in her back and hip flexors, which is due to the development of arthritis in those areas and from previous injuries. When she safely and consistently keeps up with her daily workouts and stretches, she observes that she has so much more flexibility and mobility, and she's in less pain.

The more you can pay attention to how much better you feel after integrating wellness practices into your life, the more you will want to replicate that positive feeling over and over again. Who doesn't want to feel more rested, rejuvenated, physically fit, clearheaded, and energetic? Feel free to write down your own before-and-after examples of how you feel when you incorporate specific wellness practices into your life so you can refer back to them in the future. They will serve you well and inspire you to keep integrating wellness into your life, time and time again!

THE ABOVE TIPS WILL ALLOW YOU to keep progressing from being a wellness-empowered woman to a wellness-evolved woman, which, again, means that you not only value the importance of being empowered through wellness, but you consistently prioritize your wellness in your life, day after day, even as you evolve and change. Feel free to answer the following reflection questions below so you can put a dedicated wellness plan in place.

SELF-REFLECTION QUESTIONS:

1. What does being a wellness-*empowered* woman mean to you?

2. What does being a wellness-*evolved* woman mean to you?

3. What steps can you take to stay consistent with your health and wellness regimen throughout the various stages of your life?

4. What are the biggest challenges you face now or may face in the future that impact your ability to maintain your wellness practices on a regular basis?

5. How can you shift your mindset, approach, and overall wellness plan to account for these challenges?

CHAPTER 2

WHAT IT MEANS TO LIVE A PASSION FIT LIFE THROUGH DIFFERENT LIFE STAGES

AFTER A DECADE OF BUILDING a health and wellness concept, brand, and company called Passion Fit, the Passion Fit lifestyle has become ingrained into my daily habits, perspective, and way of life. My core focus within my work has been to help my clients, students, and customers do the same.

The motto of Passion Fit is: "Pursue your passions, be fit (mentally, physically, emotionally, and spiritually), and the rest will follow." The first phase, which is what we focused on in *The Wellness-Empowered Woman*, was to figure out how to become empowered to incorporate your passions into your personal and professional life, build personalized wellness practices into your daily life, and trust that the outcome of these efforts will be favorable.

In *The Wellness-Evolved Woman,* we focus on the next phase, which is to continue living a Passion Fit life, as defined by the motto, through various stages. The key question to ask yourself is: How do I bring a level of consistency into my life so I can thrive personally and professionally, regardless of my age, circumstances, or stage in life?

The most important factor is motivation. In fact, motivation is the foundation. You have to truly want to make the effort to take care of yourself on an ongoing basis in order to sustain a healthy lifestyle in the long run. Yet, even with the best of intentions, you can sometimes hit a wall and find it difficult to stay on a healthy path. At those times, it's essential to recognize that you are human and to give yourself grace.

Everyone hits a wall at some point or another, whether it's within their wellness practices, career, or relationships. I work with clients who truly want to make or sustain healthy changes in their lives, but life just gets busy and often blocks them from sticking to their goals. Remember, it doesn't have to be all or nothing. Those are the times to take little steps, which will add up over time and can become sustainable. The key is to continue to motivate yourself and keep coming back to your goals over and over again.

A few of my long-term clients who have been a part of the Passion Fit community for years have had career changes, injuries, health issues, family transitions, and more. For example, one of my clients has been dealing with endometriosis. Along with her own physical condition, she has been tending to health issues with her parents. She also took a step back from work while preparing with her husband for their son to go off to college. Even though she has a lot on her plate, she does her best to keep up with everyone's needs as she prioritizes her own. She still pursues her passions, participating with her book club each month, and makes time to do light yoga and takes walks with her husband, son, and friends a few times per week. She's a wonderful example of someone who's living a Passion Fit life even through challenges and various stages of her life.

I've also enjoyed seeing family members benefit from living a Passion Fit life, including my parents, in-laws, siblings, cousins, and even my own husband and kids. What are some ways you can live a Passion Fit life through different stages? Read on to find out.

Take stock of your passions every few years: For some people, passions begin at a very young age and sustain themselves throughout a lifetime. For others, passions may come and go or new ones may show up at various stages of life. Taking stock of your passions will allow you to determine if the original ones are still serving you or if new passions are emerging. These passions may relate to your personal or professional life and could be part of a hobby, side hustle, or career.

Regardless of what category they fall into, having passions in your life throughout various stages can continue to infuse joy, excitement, adventure, purpose, and fulfillment into your life. So, if you love travel, music, dance, fitness, art, technology, writing, tennis, soccer, golf, nature, volunteering for a specific cause, or something else, allow your passions to come through your life at any stage. They will greatly contribute to your overall health, happiness, and well-being throughout your life!

Be aware of how your physical health is impacted during various stages: Many physical changes happen throughout life. Some examples include changes in height, hormones, reproductive system, metabolism, digestive system, allergies, hair, skin, bone density, balance, eyesight, and hearing. It's important to pay attention to these changes and proactively address them with your doctor if they present any concerns. Making sure you're eating properly, exercising regularly, and getting sufficient sleep can help as well.

As you move through life, you may need or want to make changes within those wellness practices, such as the types of foods you eat, the exercises you engage in, and the amount of sleep that suits your body during different phases. For example, higher-intensity exercises may suit your body in your twenties, thirties, and forties, but perhaps you may need to switch to lower-intensity exercises, which will most likely be easier on your joints and help you avoid injury as you get into your fifties and beyond. Another example relates to what you eat. While you may prefer animal-based proteins early in your life, perhaps post-pregnancy or in other stages of life, you may prefer plant-based proteins. Living a Passion Fit life allows you to be fit physically in ways that are appropriate for your life stage and age.

Be cognizant of how your mental health is impacted during various stages: Life can bring on both exciting moments and difficult ones, which can create positive and negative impacts on mental health. Whether it's starting a new job, getting married, having a baby, making career transitions, buying or selling a house, enduring financial hardships, or anything else, it's important to assess what's happening with your mental health. Big life changes can bring on stress, excitement, fear, and uncertainty. You may experience feelings of loss for chapters that are ending, such as a career transition or selling a house, and feelings of anticipation for new chapters that are just beginning, such as getting married or having a baby. These are all normal human emotions, so it's important to stay present and allow yourself the opportunity to process any emotions you may be feeling during each stage.

Pay attention to anxiety, depression, a lack of motivation, or any other changes as well. Seek support and address them as much as possible by talking to others and engaging in mindfulness practices, such as meditation and breathwork. For instance, take a few minutes to do diaphragmatic breathing and positive visualization. Take deep breaths and inhale through your nose while expanding out your belly, then exhale through your nose or mouth as you pull your belly back in. While you're breathing, think about a vacation destination, a loved one, or a previous memory that brings you a sense of peace, joy, and calmness.

These mindfulness practices can be used any time you need them to help protect your mental health during life transitions. In order to be resilient and mentally fit throughout your Passion Fit life, being self-aware and proactive can help you fully enjoy those joyful events and deal with the challenging ones in the healthiest manner possible.

Take note of how your emotional health is impacted during various stages: Emotional changes inevitably happen throughout the journey of life. Impacts to the brain and our social and emotional development occur during childhood and adolescence. Even as we get older, our relationship with others and ourselves can change. For instance, when we're in our adolescent years, hormonal changes can cause a wide range of emotions, including anger, euphoria, anxiety, sadness, and mood swings. These emotions can impact our personal relationships with our parents, siblings, and friends. As we move through adulthood, our emotions are often calmer and more stable, due to gained wisdom, life experiences, and self-awareness. During the pregnancy and menopausal years, our hormones shift and change again, causing an onset of heightened emotions in different situations and with different people in our lives. Due to these hormonal shifts, we might be laughing one minute and crying the next! Sometimes we don't even realize these changes are happening, and they can sneak up on us. Being tuned into ourselves and others and having a sense of emotional intelligence through journaling, healthy communication, active listening, and empathy can help us positively navigate ever-changing feelings and emotions throughout our life so we can feel good about ourselves and keep our relationships intact.

Be mindful of how your spiritual health is impacted during various stages: Spirituality looks different for everyone. Regardless of your faith or religion, belief in a higher power, or connection to the universe, it's important to be mindful of your spiritual health and what works best in your life. As life evolves and changes and both positive and negative situations occur, determining how your own spirituality can help guide you through life's complexities is a gift you can give yourself.

My faith is extremely important to me, and it's central to being able to live my life with resilience, grace, and hope. When beloved family members or friends have passed away, or I have faced uncertainties in my career or personal life, my faith has served me well by giving me strength and wisdom when I've needed it most. My faith has also allowed me to have perspective and gratitude for my life, relationships, home, and work. This is another philosophy of living a Passion Fit life, and I encourage you to deepen or find a source of spirituality that works for you.

Continue to have trust that the rest will follow and things will work out favorably: When you continue to evaluate your passions, stay fit physically, mentally, emotionally, and spiritually, even as life gives you both the expected and unexpected, having a sense of trust in the outcome is key to living a Passion Fit life. At the end of the day, it's about focusing on what we can control and letting go of what's out of our control. There's a clear sense of peace and security that can come with both taking action and letting go.

It can take time, patience, a lot of trial and error, and wisdom to arrive at this point, but it will be well worth it if you can. Remember, living a Passion Fit life and being a wellness-evolved woman is a journey and not a single destination. If you believe and trust in your own journey and take care of yourself physically, mentally, emotionally, and spiritually every step of the way, this way of living will be there for you again and again throughout the evolution of your life.

NOW THAT WE'VE REVIEWED what it means to live a Passion Fit life through different stages, take a few moments to write out your thoughts by answering the following reflection questions.

SELF-REFLECTION QUESTIONS:

1. What does living a Passion Fit life through various stages look like for you?

2. How will you assess your physical health throughout your life?

3. How will you assess your mental and emotional health throughout your life?

4. How will you assess your spiritual health throughout your life?

5. How will you maintain trust that the rest will follow and that life will eventually work out favorably for you?

CHAPTER 3

THE RELATIONSHIPS BETWEEN SELF-LOVE AND SELF-CARE

WE OFTEN HEAR ABOUT THE CONCEPT of self-care in books, magazines, movies, TV, and social media. According to Danielle Wade and Rachel Ann Tee-Melegrito, in an article featured in *Medical News Today*, seven in ten Americans are aware of their need for self-care.[2]

Self-care is the regular practice of taking care of our mental, physical, and emotional health through activities such as taking a bath, reading a good book, drinking a cup of tea, stretching, taking a walk, talking to a loved one or friend or writing in a journal. But in this busy, modern world, we're constantly connected to technology, which can often make it difficult to unplug and make time for self-care. It can also be challenging to communicate our need to take a break and practice self-care with those in our personal and professional lives because we often focus on others' needs at the expense of our own. Yet, as stated above, most people recognize the need for and the importance of self-care.

And while self-care is extremely important for maintaining our sense of health and well-being, it needs to start with a true sense of self-love. Only then will we actually prioritize ourselves and our self-care. Self-love isn't meant to be egotistical or self-centered. It's a critical part of living an authentic and healthy life. One of the most important relationships we have in life is the one we have with ourselves. It's the root of all our other relationships. If we can't love ourselves, how can we love anyone else?

When we are young, we usually have a very pure sense of self-love and love for others. As we get older, life situations, experiences, and external messages can often affect our sense of self-love. For example, if we struggle or fail at something, receive negative feedback from someone in our personal or professional life, feel we don't live up to societal expectations, or compare ourselves to others, our self-love can be impacted.

Every stage in life can include complexities that challenge our self-love. We may not feel as if we are good enough in certain relationships, at school, in our jobs, or in other life circumstances. I've worked with clients who lack a sense of self-love and struggle with feeling confident within themselves, leaving them unable to take actions, such as stick to a fitness program, take risks in their careers, move to a new city, or try a new sport.

Confidence is a feeling linked to self-love. When you truly love yourself, including your strengths, weaknesses, and everything in between, you are more likely to be confident in your abilities. You trust that you will be able to handle situations as they come, and you will eventually succeed in your pursuits and endeavors.

According to Ana Sandoiu and Jasmin Collier in an article featured in *Medical News Today*, another deterrent to self-love is perfectionism.[3] As I shared in *The Wellness-Empowered Woman*, I've struggled with perfectionism most of my life. I am also married to a fellow perfectionist, and we tend to feed off of each other at times. The good news is I am very self-aware, and while I still have high standards, I have worked hard over the years to overcome my perfectionism and not be as hard on myself as I used to be. My husband has also put in the work and done the same. Both of our efforts in this area will also benefit our kids, who also have perfectionist tendencies ... probably because of us!

One of the most important actions we can take for our mental and emotional health is to let go of perfectionism or any other deterrents to self-love so we can find and maintain our sense of self-love throughout our lives. While this is often easier said than done, here are five practices to work toward a deeper sense of self-love.

Address the deterrents to self-love from your past and present life: Most things in life have a cause-and-effect relationship. There are usually deeper reasons behind our emotions, feelings, perceptions, and beliefs. As a result, it's important to take some time to address and understand where our perspectives come from. Were there experiences in your childhood that impacted your sense of self-love or the way you view yourself in general? As you progressed into your teenage years, were there any defining moments that impacted you? What about in your adult life? Where do you stand now in terms of your feelings of self-love?

If you are rooted in self-love and feel you have a healthy sense of it, that's great. If you struggle with self-love for various reasons, that's okay too. The key is to talk about or write out what you are feeling and why. Seeking out support from loved ones or a professional can help you with this process as well. It may not be an easy process to go through, but the internal work is well worth the effort. It can help you overcome any deterrents and help put you on the path to discovering or rediscovering your sense of self-love.

Shift your mindset toward self-love: No matter what has happened in the past or even what's happening in the present, striving to love ourselves unconditionally as we go forward into the future is important for our overall health and well-being. When we think about our family members, we love them unconditionally, right? So why shouldn't we be able to love ourselves unconditionally as well? We all have flaws because that's part of being human. However, when we come from a place of self-love, we can lead with love in other areas and with other people in our lives. Self-love can often help reduce feelings of frustration, anger, bitterness, and resentment toward ourselves and other people, places, and situations. It allows us to free ourselves of those critical and negative thoughts we may have and can allow us to have more empathy for ourselves and others.

Making a mindset shift toward self-love will take practice

and patience. One of the best ways to work on this is through mindfulness and meditation. Quiet your environment and your mind, close your eyes, and take some deep breaths from your diaphragm. Focus your thoughts on unconditional love for yourself, and if your mind wanders toward critical and negative thoughts, gently guide your thoughts back to those of self-love. The more you do this, the easier it will become, and eventually, you will be able to tap into your sense of self-love more easily and effortlessly.

Write down your favorite qualities about yourself: Another way to discover or reclaim your sense of self-love is to write down the qualities you love most about yourself. This is meant to be a personal and private writing exercise in your journal, so don't be shy! You can write about your values, personality traits, appearance, skills, education, passions, career, relationships, impact on others, faith, or anything else that comes to mind. You can also write out specific examples or stories that reflect times when you were proud of an accomplishment or the way you handled a certain situation. You could write about forgiving yourself if you handled a situation in a manner that you weren't proud of as well. What did you learn from that situation, and what might you do differently next time? Are there any other elements of your past you would like to let go of in order to feel a sense of self-love? Write it down.

Allow yourself to write freely and without judgment. Don't hold back because you probably have more qualities you respect and love about yourself than you may even realize. This is the time to jot it all down so that you can refer back to it whenever you need a pick-me-up. This writing can also serve as your true internal voice, which can replace any negative feelings you may experience in the future.

Allow family and close friends to remind you of why you are loved: In addition to working on our own self-love, it also helps to be reminded of why we are loved by those closest to us. As humans, we need relationships and social connection to survive. In fact, according to Amy Novotney, in an article featured by the *American Psychological Association*, social isolation and loneliness are as detrimental to your health as smoking or obesity.[4] In the quest for self-love, it's critical to connect with those you love and trust so you can feel loved by others, which will, in turn, help you love yourself.

Ask your parents, significant other, spouse, or others in your life what they love about you. You are not fishing for compliments; you are simply asking them to remind you and provide you with insight into what makes you loveable, especially in cases where you may have forgotten. They will more likely than not be thrilled to share what they love about you. You can also reciprocate and share what you love about them too. The silver lining of this exercise is that you may end up strengthening your relationships with others as you also strive to strengthen your relationship with yourself!

Practice ongoing compassion for yourself: Even with the best of intentions and diligent inner work, life events, circumstances, or other peoples' opinions of us can cause us to take a few steps back in our quest for self-love. That's okay and completely normal—and part of the process. Just like in life, our relationship with ourselves and our sense of self-love isn't always linear. Sometimes, it can be a zigzagging mess! But again, we are human, and the more we can anticipate that this regression might happen, the more self-aware and alert we will be, and the more we can choose our reactions and stop in their tracks, any future deterrents to self-love. The key is to practice ongoing compassion for ourselves.

We are so often taught about having compassion for others, but it's also imperative that we have it for ourselves. That compassion will be the voice of reason that will save us time and time again from dipping back into a lack of self-love and an increase in those negative emotions of self-doubt, fear, frustration, resentment, and bitterness. Like the other four practices we talked about, practicing compassion for ourselves will take repetition, time, and patience. But it's absolutely possible and can positively impact your mental and emotional health.

THIS CONCEPT OF SELF-LOVE is one of the key themes woven throughout this book. Looking back, I somehow understood the importance of self-love at a young age—it even showed up prominently in my mission statement. Even if I didn't always feel it in different periods of my life, I've always come back to it and will continue to put in the work to do so in the future. I attribute that understanding to the unconditional love I received from my parents, and I'm so incredibly grateful for that. And now as a parent myself, and in partnership with my husband, I work hard to provide that same unconditional love for our kids so they can practice self-love as well.

Self-love encompasses addressing the deterrents in your life, shifting your mindset, reflecting on your favorite qualities, giving and asking for open and honest feedback from your loved ones, and having compassion. These elements of self-love sound a lot like the elements of a successful relationship with others, don't they? That's by design, and they drive home the point that by loving ourselves, we will sincerely have the skills to love others, and vice versa. Also, by loving ourselves, we will be able to move more confidently from one life stage to another. We will have a stronger sense of self-esteem, inner security, and faith that we can take on whatever life throws our way. And hopefully, we will be able to do so with strength, humility, and grace.

NOW THAT YOU HAVE SOME PRACTICES you can leverage for discovering or rediscovering your sense of self-love, feel free to jot down some thoughts in response to the following questions.

SELF-REFLECTION QUESTIONS:

1. What does the concept of self-love mean to you?

2. Do you feel you have a healthy sense of self-love?

3. If you do have a healthy sense of self-love, why? If you don't, why not?

4. While it would be ideal to put into practice all five efforts toward finding or creating self-love, which steps would have the most impact on you and why?

5. What can you do to be more aware of any deterrents to your sense of self-love, and what can you do to stop them in their tracks?

CHAPTER 4

WHERE YOU'VE BEEN, WHERE YOU ARE, AND WHERE YOU'RE GOING

AS WE CONTINUE ALONG THE JOURNEY of becoming a wellness-evolved woman, we are going to take some time to look at where you've been, where you are, and where you're going. Specifically, we are going to look at birth order, where you grew up compared to where you live now, and your personality traits. Having insights into these areas can help us make sense of how our lives began, how they've evolved and changed since then, and what direction we might be heading in the future. Understanding these foundations can also help us apply our wellness practices to our physical, mental, emotional, and spiritual health so we can continue to navigate through the journey of life in a healthy and whole way.

Let's start with where you've been, specifically your birth order, as it's an interesting topic when it comes to wellness because it has the potential to shape our lives in many ways. How we were raised by our parents and our dynamic with our siblings as a first-born child, middle child, youngest child, or only child can impact our health and well-being, personality, tendencies, perspectives, education, career choices, and personal relationships.

As the youngest of four children and a mother of two children, I certainly have my own experiences and perspectives on this, which I will share as well. That said, every individual and family is unique and special in their own way, and birth order doesn't necessarily result in stereotypical traits or labels, but it can pop up. While the information shared in this chapter is based on research, it isn't meant to be absolute or applicable for everyone.

According to Kevin Leman, Ph.D., a psychologist and author of *The Birth Order Book: Why You Are the Way You Are*, and as featured in a June 26, 2023, *Parents Magazine* article, parents may knowingly and unknowingly treat their children differently based on birth order.[5] For example, they may be more strict, structured, and hyper-focused with their first-born child and more relaxed, unstructured, and divided with their attention with subsequent children.

Birth order can also influence each child's position in the family and relationship with their siblings, as noted by Meri Wallace, a child and family therapist and author of *Birth Order Blues*.[6] For example, sibling dynamics can present themselves, such as being a leader or a follower, being more or less vocal, and being more or less responsible. Research shows the following potential characteristics within each position in a family.

First-born children may be given a lot of responsibility and have high expectations placed upon them by their parents to set a good example for their younger siblings. They inevitably experience different stages of life before their siblings and may require a lot of attention and focus from their parents. Sometimes, the focus from parents can be overwhelming since parents may carry the stress of going through these stages for the first time along with their oldest child.

Middle children can be the peacekeepers between their older and younger siblings. Their parents may not always be as attentive as they would like because they are focused on the older and younger siblings, sometimes leaving middle children to feel somewhat lost in the family dynamics. That said, some parents might be aware of this tendency and may make the extra effort to help their middle children feel heard, understood, and included. Middle children may also want to differentiate themselves from their older and younger siblings, and as a result, may have different interests, likes, dislikes, and styles compared to their other siblings.

Younger children may initially require extra attention compared to their older siblings because they simply need more help in the early stages. Parents and older siblings may "baby" the younger ones and older siblings may even tease them. That being said, some younger children may be more independent and outgoing because they are used to being around other children, and their parents might be more relaxed after parenting the siblings who came before them, and there may be less oversight, rules, and restrictions. Younger children may also already know what to expect in various situations through watching their older siblings' experiences, potentially making them more confident.

Only children may be used to getting full attention from their parents. They don't have any siblings with whom they have to share, nor do they have any siblings with whom they could have conflicts. Only children may potentially feel lonely at times, especially when comparing their home life to their friends or relatives who have siblings, or perhaps they don't feel lonely, since they don't know any different but do spend more time alone.

As mentioned, these dynamics and characteristics may vary from family to family and from child to child. As the youngest child, I know I felt a mix of these. Sometimes, I felt I received a lot of attention, help, and babying by everyone in my family when I was younger. However, my parents were also sometimes more relaxed with me than they were with my older siblings, allowing me space and independence. Also, I often felt confident in situations since I'd watched my brothers and sister go through them before I did. I also experienced some friendly teasing from my siblings, which sometimes made me more sensitive, sometimes made me tougher, and sometimes helped me to have a sense of humor.

Overall, my birth order has certainly played a role in my quest to become a wellness-evolved woman. I've tried to channel all the love I've received from my family throughout my life into my own self-love and care for my health and well-being, as well as take the wisdom and learnings I've gained from my parents and siblings to embrace change throughout my life. I've also tried to be cognizant of my upbringing and how I integrate it into parenting my own children.

Both my husband and I try to remain self-aware of our parenting styles, even if we parent somewhat differently between our older and younger sons. For example, we tend to look to our older son as a role model for our younger son, given they have similar academic and athletic interests. And we were not as stressed with our younger son when we went through different stages of childhood, and now his teenage years, as we were with our older son because we've already been through them once before, albeit with a different personality previously. We try to respect their differences and be fair and equal in our love and focus on each of them. We are certainly not perfect, but we try our best and keep learning and growing, as my parents did with my siblings and me.

Take a moment here to consider your birth order. Did your birth order impact your life in certain ways? Did the way in which you were parented as a result of your birth order impact your life as well? If so, how? Do you see any correlations between your birth order and your behavioral approach to your health and well-being? For example, do you take responsibility for your health and wellness with proactive lifestyle choices? Do you follow what others are doing or look for others to direct your approach to your health and well-being? Or do you march to the beat of your own drum when it comes to your health and wellness, creating something that is unique to you?

It's always beneficial to have an awareness of ourselves as individuals, as well as how our family dynamics have impacted us. This level of awareness can help as we strive to strengthen our relationship with ourselves and others. As wellness-evolved women, we may even find that although our birth order played a role in our upbringing, we can create a whole new approach to the way we choose to live.

Let's focus next on where you grew up compared to where you live now. Do you still live in the geographic area where you grew up or, upon becoming an adult, did you move elsewhere for college, graduate school, or work? Whether you've stayed in your hometown or moved away, where you grew up can often have a lifelong influence on you and your perspective in life.

According to Brian Knop and Lydia Anderson in the September 9, 2020, *United States Census Bureau* article, over one-third of married couples still live in the same state where they both were born.[7]

My husband and I are actually from the same state of Wisconsin, our hometowns are only thirty minutes away from one another in the suburbs of Milwaukee, and we went to the same college in Madison. However, we didn't meet until a few years after college, when we were both living in San Francisco.

Even though my husband and I met in California, we have a lot in common because we were both born and raised in the Midwest. Where we grew up was one of the commonalities that instantly drew us to each other. We share similar values when it comes to being down to earth, valuing hard work, treating others with genuine kindness, caring about our community, and being resilient. And as a result of living in a few different cities and states across the country and traveling domestically and internationally together before settling down in San Diego, we've expanded our perspectives and life experiences beyond where we grew up.

That being said, marrying or dating someone who grew up in a different geographic location can also be fulfilling. You have the opportunity to learn so much about each other's respective cities, states, or countries. There's a richness and depth that can permeate your relationship and instill growth as a couple and individually.

Living in a different location from where you grew up can also expand your horizons and open your eyes to new experiences and ways of living. And if you live in the same town where you grew up, you can still find opportunities for growth when you travel and visit other places. Always remember: the place where you grew up is evolving and changing as well.

Overall, the life experiences you have, regardless of where you've lived, can have a huge impact on who you were, who you are, and who you will become. In an effort to become a wellness-evolved woman, taking some time to reflect on these aspects of life can help in your self-understanding and self-compassion.

Let's now focus on personality and how it factors into becoming a wellness-evolved woman. We are going to explore how your personality traits impact your health and wellness, as well as your personal and professional development.

According to Jing Luo, Bo Zhang, and Daniel K. Mroczek in the June 21, 2022, article featured in the *Society for Personality and Social Psychology*, there has been a long-standing link between personality traits and health, as positive developments over time in personality traits, such as openness and conscientiousness, can result in health improvements.[8]

When you consider yourself, how do you describe your personality? How do others describe your personality?

There are many personality tests out there, and two of the top tests, according to Hallie Crawford, in a July 30, 2021, article in *U.S. News & World Report* include Myers-Briggs and Enneagram.[9] I've taken Myers-Briggs a few different times, and I have many colleagues who've taken Enneagram. From a behavioral and psychological perspective, they each have their unique focuses and differentiators.

Let's take a look at these two tests and how they can be applied to our lives.

Myers-Briggs: With over seventy years of science and research-based insights, the Myers-Briggs personality test is a comprehensive tool for self-awareness and self-improvement. It focuses on where you draw your energy from (extraversion versus introversion), how you receive and analyze information (sensing versus intuition), how you draw conclusions (thinking versus feeling), and how you approach life in the outside world (judging versus perceiving). All of these elements directly relate to your health, happiness, and well-being as well.

I've taken this test several times, and I consistently present as an ENFJ, which stands for: extraversion (draws energy from being with people and outside experiences), intuition (builds associations and focuses on possibilities), feeling (approaches situations using human values and motives) and judging (lives life in a planned and organized way). I definitely see the ways these attributes impact how I approach my career, family, friendships, home, community, and mindset.

I've always been an extrovert. I love to be around family and friends and to meet new people as well. I highly value my personal and professional relationships and invest a great deal of time and energy into them. I'm an intuitive person and use my intuition, which is based on previous and present experiences and information, to make decisions for the future. I'm also in touch with my feelings and live my life according to my core and human values. In addition, I prioritize expressing my feelings through written and verbal communication with others. Finally, I'm a type-A personality and like to be organized, as it helps reduce stress and makes me feel calm and in control.

I highly recommend taking this test if you haven't already, as it will provide you with many insights into yourself as well.

Enneagram: This personality assessment focuses on how emotions drive your life and how you interact with others to get what you need and want in life. There are nine personality types, including the reformer, helper, achiever, individualist, investigator, loyalist, enthusiast, challenger, and peacemaker. These personality types fall under three key categories of body types, head types, and heart types. This assessment is a great way to understand what motivates you on a deep level so you can create a path to self-actualization. You will also be able to tune into your emotional health and understand how your personality traits and emotions impact your relationship with yourself and others.

TAKING THE TIME TO GO DEEP into your past, present, and potential future can allow you to connect with and understand yourself. This type of inner work can also go a long way in becoming a wellness-evolved woman. When you're able to reflect upon and love your true and most authentic self, based on all the chapters of your life you've already lived, you will most likely want to continue to take even better care of yourself so you can make the most out of the rest of your life's journey, both personally and professionally. After exploring birth order, where you grew up compared to where you live now, and personality traits, take some time to apply your learnings and answer the following reflection questions below.

SELF-REFLECTION QUESTIONS:

1. What is your birth order, and how do you think it impacts your life today?

2. How have the locations where you grew up and where you live now impacted your views and perspectives?

3. What are your core personality traits, and have they always been there or have they changed and evolved over time?

4. How can you take your learnings about where you were, where you are now, and where you want to go and apply them to your health and well-being?

5. How has your past impacted your present, and how might your past and present impact your future?

CHAPTER 5

EMBRACING CHANGE, OUR ONLY CONSTANT IN LIFE

THE CONCEPT OF CHANGE can be multifaceted. In some instances, change can feel exhilarating and refreshing. In other instances, it can feel daunting and scary. Regardless of how change can feel, it's inevitable and necessary.

As wellness-evolved women, the more we can embrace change in all its forms, the better off we will be from a mental and emotional health standpoint because change is our only constant in life. This is one of the key distinctions from going from a wellness-empowered woman to a wellness-evolved one. When we become empowered through wellness, we may find ourselves challenged by changes that occur during a specific moment in time or stage in our life or for a specific reason. When we become evolved through wellness, we understand that change will undoubtedly occur throughout the many stages of our lives. As wellness-evolved women, we open ourselves to the possibilities offered through change.

In August 2020, during the pandemic, my family and I decided to drive from Silicon Valley to San Diego to shelter in place with my parents for a few weeks. We wanted to spend time with them before the kids started virtual school in the fall, and we needed a change of scenery after being stuck at home that summer.

A few hours after we arrived, as we sat outside in the backyard with my parents, my mom suggested we look at model homes while we were in town. While I had always wanted to live in Southern California long term, and my husband and I had talked in the past about moving from Northern to Southern California at some point in the future when the kids went to college and we retired, we certainly weren't thinking about moving in the middle of a pandemic and were both surprised by the suggestion.

My parents explained that they had always hoped all of their children and grandchildren would live in one place someday, but especially now, since the pandemic had created so much uncertainty. Since my parents had just moved from Milwaukee to San Diego a few years earlier, and my siblings and their families had already been living in San Diego, Orange County, and Los Angeles for many years by that point as well, my parents were hoping we would join all of them.

My husband and I understood where they were coming from, and the pandemic certainly did cause us to rethink our priorities. Family had always been our number one priority, and we also loved San Diego. However, after living in the Bay

Area for twenty years, we were concerned about the impacts on my husband's job at Google, my business, our community of friends, and our kids' attachment to their friends, schools, and sports teams, especially since we were living in such unprecedented times. We weren't sure if more change would be detrimental or beneficial.

Nonetheless, we got curious and looked online at new home developments in San Diego. We came across a beautiful development that caught our eye. The next day, I suggested to my husband that we go with my parents and the kids to take a look. My husband didn't expect me to be serious about moving. I told him I thought we should keep an open mind and check it out. Nervously, he agreed. As soon as we entered the new home development, I was giddy with excitement. It was such a beautiful area and neighborhood, and the model homes were gorgeous. I had a strong intuitive feeling that this would be our future and long-term home. We then spoke to one of the salespeople, toured the model homes, and were given some paperwork indicating which home lots were still available, as well as pricing and building timelines.

After gathering all the information and talking to my family, I said to my husband that if he and the kids were up for moving, I would do it in a heartbeat. Although he loved the new home development too and wanted to live closer to family, he was understandably concerned about the impacts on his job and wanted to talk to his boss first. We also were met with resistance from our kids, who were understandably in shock and confused as to how a trip to San Diego to visit their grandparents suddenly turned into us potentially deciding to move there.

Because only four home lots were left in the neighborhood, and they were selling fast, we had about a week to make a decision. That week felt like the longest week ever. Thankfully, my husband's boss was supportive of the move. His only request was that my husband travel up to Google headquarters twice a month to stay connected to the team, which made sense. My husband and I then had some serious conversations about a major life and financial decision, and we also tried to help our kids feel more comfortable about the decision as well.

In the end, we all decided that moving to San Diego to be closer to our extended family was the best decision for us. And now, about three years later, I can honestly say my husband, kids, and I are all thriving and incredibly happy. My kids love their schools, sports teams, and friends; my husband's job is going extremely well; my business is successful and growing; and we have made so many wonderful friends here. And living near the beach and mountains is amazing. Most importantly, we love living near our family for support in good or challenging times, and for the opportunity to create precious memories over major milestones, holidays, and simple, everyday moments as well.

This story is an example of embracing change as a wellness-evolved woman. When faced with the move, my mindset was immediately one of curiosity and openness to possibility, instead of feeling resistant to change. I was able to look at all the ways our family could benefit from the move instead of feeling threatened by it. And thankfully, I was able to help my family shift to that mindset as well. My ability to embrace change has certainly come with years of experience, but even when change scared me in my youth, I still moved toward it instead of away from it. I have always sought to explore and be open to new ideas, people, and experiences.

EVEN THOUGH CHANGE CAN be uncomfortable and challenging, there can be so much joy, growth, happiness, and adventure on the other side of it. Life is a journey, and as humans, we are meant to experience new things. This can apply to many aspects of life, including changes to where we live, where we work, and where we travel. It can take time to first process and work through changes, whether big or small, because they can impact us in both the short term and long term, as well as personally and professionally, but the end result may turn out to be even more wondrous than we imagined!

In becoming a wellness-evolved woman, you are able to look at change from a wider lens filled with perspective, wisdom, and courage. Placing your personal wellness at the center of change can allow you to think through it with a clear mind and an open heart, especially if you are nourishing your mind, body, and spirit with proper sleep, meditation, deep breathing, healthy food, and movement. You will gain the strength and resilience to embrace the change by taking care of your physical, mental, emotional, and spiritual health first.

I work with many corporate clients on employee wellness, and over the last few years, there has been a significant amount of change in the workplace. From many companies asking employees to work virtually 100 percent of the time during the pandemic, to some companies now requiring employees back in the office full time, to other companies taking a hybrid approach and offering both in-office and remote work, to layoffs and cost cutting due to a looming recession, people have been experiencing change in abundance in their professional lives since the start of this decade.

These changes can also have an effect on people's personal lives because their work lives impact their home lives, and vice versa. People often have to rethink their commutes, childcare, work travel, and other daily logistics. These changes have had a massive impact on employee health and well-being. In fact, according to a State of the Workplace Global Report from *Gallup* in 2023, employee stress has remained at a record high, causing 44 percent of surveyed employees to experience substantial stress on a daily basis.[10] I've seen this level of stress firsthand with employees of companies I've spoken to and consulted with, especially in recent years. Employees have shared with me their experiences of anxiety and burnout, given all the moving parts in their lives. This level of stress has become far too common in our society, which is a cause for concern and an indicator of the need for intentional action.

It's essential to protect our health from stress that can often come with change so it doesn't lead to bigger issues down the road. This is an important part of my work with both individual and corporate clients, and I feel very strongly about creating wellness tools and educating others on how to use them.

If you are experiencing stress as a result of personal or professional changes in your life, here are four actions you can take on a regular basis to deal with change as it comes. **Understand why the change is causing discomfort:** Oftentimes, you feel stressed about a change but don't know what the reasoning is behind it. It's important to take the time to understand why you're feeling discomfort through activities such as journaling, talking to a professional, or engaging in other forms of self-reflection. Consider questions such as: Will the change impact your relationships, health, job, home, finances, security, livelihood, or something else? The more you can uncover about the change and its impact on your life, the more you will understand it and feel prepared and equipped to deal with it. While it isn't always easy to delve into what makes you uncomfortable, the more you do it each time you experience change, the stronger you become and the less scary it will be over time.

Shift your mindset to view the change as an opportunity for growth instead of a threat: Even when change can cause disruption in your life, whether it's moving to a new city, starting a new job or business, beginning or ending a relationship, creating a change in behavior for better health, or changing your lifestyle due to a new life stage, having the right mindset can go a long way to make the change easier to deal with. No matter what the change may be and how hard it might be to manage it in the beginning, you will undoubtedly learn and grow from it. When you can shift your mindset to one of curiosity and openness and view the change as an opportunity for learning and growth instead of a threat, it can actually become a positive instead of a negative occurrence in your life. Mindset is everything, and it's amazing how a shift in perspective can be the difference between thriving versus surviving through changes in your life.

Mentally prepare for the best-case and worst-case scenarios that could arise from the change: Even when you try to stay positive, fears, negative feelings, or challenging outcomes can come from change as well, even if they are temporary. So, in order to be resilient through change, try to prepare mentally for the best-case and worst-case scenarios. What's the best and worst thing that could happen? How might you feel? How might a positive outcome enhance your life, and how might you deal with a negative outcome in the best possible way? How will both positive and negative outcomes bring on stress in some form, and how will you deal with that stress? If you take the time to sort through these potential feelings and outcomes, you will feel prepared because you have already thought about them and have a plan in place. And even if the outcome ends up being completely different from what you had anticipated, the mental preparation will allow you to take on courageously whatever comes your way.

Embrace the change with confidence and take action: Once you've thought through why a change might cause you discomfort, shifted your mindset to view it as an opportunity as opposed to a threat, and mentally prepared for the best-case and worst-case scenarios, you're ready to embrace change with confidence and take action. Again, change is our only constant in life, so the more we can anticipate and prepare for it, the more we can move through it with courage, minimize our stress levels, and ultimately protect our mental and physical health and well-being. While this process may take some time, it's one of the most important skills we can learn in life. One of the cornerstones of being a wellness-evolved woman is handling change with openness, curiosity, strength, wisdom, resilience, and grace!

IT'S NOW TIME TO PUT THESE CONCEPTS into practice and apply them to your own life.

Feel free to answer the following reflection questions below, which you can refer back to any time you're experiencing change in the future.

SELF-REFLECTION QUESTIONS:

1. Are you currently experiencing any changes in your life?

2. Are these changes causing you to feel any kind of stress or discomfort, possibly impacting your physical or mental health negatively?

3. If you are feeling stress or discomfort, why do you think that might be?

4. How can you shift your mindset and view these changes as opportunities to learn and grow?

5. What are the best and worst things that can happen, and how can you embrace the changes and move through them with confidence and resilience?

CHAPTER 6

ETHNICITY AND AUTHENTICITY GO HAND IN HAND

BEING BORN AND RAISED IN WISCONSIN as a first-generation Indian-American in the late seventies, eighties, and nineties was an interesting experience that profoundly impacted my life. The US, especially in the Midwest, wasn't as diversely populated at that time as it is today. And even today, there's much more diversity on the East and West Coasts compared to the Midwest.

While we did have a small community of family friends who we saw occasionally on the weekends, who were immigrant parents from India with first-generation Indian-American children, I often felt different in my daily life from my Caucasian friends and peers in my school, neighborhood, and extracurricular activities. Back then, I so badly wanted to fit in and be American like everyone else, especially when kids in school asked me a lot of questions about my ethnicity or poked fun at me for being different.

While it's hard for me to admit now, I often felt embarrassed that my family spoke Hindi in addition to English; listened to Bollywood music in addition to the top 40 songs playing on the radio; ate chicken curry, rice, naan, and saag paneer for dinner more than pizza, burgers, chicken casserole, or pasta; meditated, did yoga, and went to the Hindu temple instead of church; and wore brightly colored and embellished Indian clothes for special occasions, such as Diwali, Holi, family weddings, or holiday folk fairs. It's not that I didn't like these aspects of our culture—deep down, I really did—I just felt uncomfortable sharing them with my American friends because I worried about being judged or not accepted. In college, I even wrote a paper called, *Indian or American: Caught Between Two Cultures.* I often felt I wasn't Indian enough with my Indian friends, and I wasn't American enough with my American friends.

Noticing my embarrassment and discomfort during my younger years, my parents often said to me, "No matter where you go or what you do, people won't let you forget who you are or where you come from, so embrace it and be proud of it." Those were powerful words that have stuck with me throughout my life. And looking back, I am so glad they taught me this very important lifelong lesson. Many times in life, we try to be someone we are not or hide parts of ourselves for fear of not fitting in. But in the end, it will be to our detriment. The sooner we can realize this, the better.

As for me, fast forward a few decades later. The very

aspects of my ethnic identity that had caused me so much embarrassment and discomfort when I was younger are the aspects of who I am that I'm now most proud of and want to celebrate and instill in my children. I came to these realizations due to my life experiences, meeting and becoming friends with a more diverse group of people, including more fellow Indians, and feeling more social acceptance of different cultures in society today. And what I didn't realize then is that ethnicity and authenticity go hand in hand. Those elements of my rich and beautiful Indian culture that made me feel different when I was younger are so incredibly special and distinctive and will forever be a part of who I am.

Another defining moment in my journey to embrace my ethnic identity is when I was preparing to marry my husband, who is not Indian and is Caucasian. In Indian culture, you are usually expected to marry someone of the same or similar background, as that has been the custom over many centuries. In my case, my soulmate in life ended up not being Indian, but someone who completely embraced my Indian culture from day one. He's always loved Indian food, Indian music, and Bollywood movies, and even had his own set of Indian friends before he met me. My family loves him dearly, and they jokingly call him practically Indian, since he's been married into an Indian family for *over* twenty years.

I will never forget an important conversation my husband and I had a few weeks before our wedding. Since I wasn't marrying someone Indian, I was feeling emotional and worried about losing a part of my Indian identity, which I'd begun to discover and embrace. When I vulnerably opened up to him about this fear, he lovingly said, "Keep going down the path of discovering this part of yourself, and I'll follow you." His sweet words brought me to tears, and it's one of the most wonderfully encouraging statements he's ever said to me. I needed to hear those words in that moment, and what they made me realize was that meeting him had ironically played a big role in me finally embracing my Indian identity. He helped me appreciate it and see it through his fresh eyes. What a gift! And I love that we are raising our half-Indian boys to love and appreciate both their Indian and American identities as well.

AS I DID RESEARCH FOR THIS BOOK on the impact of ethnicity on wellness, I came across many scholarly articles related to the social determinants of health and how people of different ethnic backgrounds experience adverse outcomes in their physical and mental health. The causes are mainly due to inequalities in access to health care, varying socioeconomic backgrounds, and racism. These are unfortunate realities many people have to face, and much more work needs to be done to create greater equity in our society. Through education, volunteer work, and donations, I will continue to do my part to help those in need.

For purposes of this book, I want to look at ethnicity through a different lens. What if we all embraced our cultural identities and those of others early on, or at any stage in life, for the purposes of increasing our mental and emotional health, authenticity, self-esteem, self-love, love for others, empathy, and unity? How powerful would that be?! Research shows there is a correlation between strong ethnic identities and quality of life, well-being, and self-confidence. Even if you are several generations removed from your ethnic origin, there is still so much exploration and discovery that can happen. Taking the time to assess this part of yourself and others can allow for learning, growth, and self-awareness, which can be quite enriching. Here are four ways embracing your ethnicity and those of others can positively impact your life.

Social connection: In addition to having a diverse group of friends, also being able to connect with others who have similar backgrounds, family traditions, and languages can create a strong sense of community and social support. It's important to have others in your social circle who are like-minded, who you can relate to, and who can relate to you. Social connections and wellness go hand in hand because humans are naturally social creatures. We are meant to connect with others, and our health and well-being actually depend on it. According to the *Centers for Disease Control* in a March 30, 2023, article, social connection is deeply personal, and each individual must determine how to seek and nurture meaningful relationships throughout their lives to optimize their mental and emotional health.[11] We will talk more about social connections in Chapter Nine.

Enhanced perspective: Different cultures have different perspectives when it comes to marriage, family, education, careers, finances, health, well-being, customs, and beliefs. Connecting with your own cultural identity and that of others can allow you to enhance your personal perspective on many of these topics, especially if you were born and raised in a different country than that of your origin. It's also a way to feel connected to your relatives and ancestors. You can benefit from intergenerational perspectives as well. I know I've greatly benefited from the perspectives of my grandparents, parents, aunts, uncles, and cousins, many of whom were born and raised in India. Throughout my life, they've offered a different way of looking at various situations, which has expanded my mind and heart. Consider how you can connect to those parts of your family history and lineage as well.

Sense of belonging: Connecting with our own culture or the culture of others in our life can also provide a sense of belonging and feeling a part of something bigger than ourselves. In a world where so much of our time is spent using technology, which can be isolating, focusing on in-person connection with our families, friends, and communities, including those who share our ethnicity, can be refreshing and energizing. A sense of belonging can especially be felt during holidays, family celebrations, and cultural observances. Being fully present during these special occasions can be extremely fulfilling and allow us to create memories that will last a lifetime.

Positive identity: Life can be complex, and certain life stages can cause us to feel lost, especially when we are experiencing change. Connecting with the deeper parts of ourselves, including our ethnicities, can create a positive identity. It can allow us to understand who we are and where we come from, which can be especially comforting in challenging times and times of change. Even if we haven't embraced our ethnicity in the past, we can connect to it and embody it at any time. The choice is ours, and it's never too late. And having a positive identity can also contribute to higher self-esteem and self-love. These are *all* ingredients for becoming a wellness-evolved woman.

Wellness is holistic and spans across our physical, mental, emotional, and spiritual health. And ethnicity is genuinely connected to all of these aspects of wellness because it's an important part of the fabric that makes up who we authentically are—from our physical features, to our viewpoints, to our relationships, to our customs, to our beliefs. Times have changed over the last several decades, and where it once was more desirable to assimilate and conform to be like everyone else, we are now living in a time where authenticity and uniqueness are more encouraged and celebrated. While we still have a long way to go, this is a huge progression from when I was growing up. And I'm happy that future generations, which include my kids, will be able to connect to this part of themselves more openly and freely.

I HOPE THIS CHAPTER HAS ALLOWED YOU to consider a whole new dimension to your wellness. If your ethnicity has been a source of stress or confusion in the past, I encourage you to take the necessary steps to gain more clarity. And if you haven't spent too much time exploring your ethnicity, I invite you to give it consideration in the present and future. In order to explore your ethnicity and authenticity further, feel free to answer the following self-reflection questions listed below. Whether you are first-generation American like

I am or a few generations removed, your cultural roots are worth exploring, especially as you continue down the path of becoming a wellness-evolved woman.

SELF-REFLECTION QUESTIONS:

1. Are you currently connected to your ethnicity?

2. If so, how are you connected, and if not, why not?

3. What role, if any, has your ethnicity played in your life over the years?

4. Does your ethnicity impact your identity, authenticity, health, and well-being, and if so, how?

5. Would you like to continue to explore your cultural identity to more deeply connect with yourself, your family, and your ancestry, and if so, what steps can you take to start doing so?

CHAPTER 7

INNATE TALENTS, STRENGTHS, AND SKILLS: A BLUEPRINT FOR SUCCESS

ACCORDING TO A 2023 ARTICLE in *Gallup,* people who take the CliftonStrengths assessment and have the opportunity to leverage their strengths at work are six times more likely to be engaged in their jobs, six times more likely to feel they are able to do what they're best at every day, and six times more likely to have an excellent quality of life.[12] Each of us has our unique mix of strengths because, according to Jim Asplund and within research featured in the November 5, 2021, article in *Gallup,* the chances of any two people having the same top five strengths are one in thirty-three million.[13]

Over the last two decades, while I worked at Yahoo, Google, and now Passion Fit, I've taken the Gallup CliftonStrengths course, read the book, and completed the assessment to better understand my innate talents, strengths, and skills. In the three times I've taken this assessment, my top five to ten strengths have remained relatively the same, which, to me, validates the accuracy of this assessment and the fact that my strengths are truly innate. I've also been able to see how my strengths have played out in various stages of my life, from my early to mid-careers, marriage to motherhood, and everything in between.

My top ten strengths from the assessment include the following:

- Achiever
- Discipline
- Focus
- Woo (connecting with people)
- Positivity
- Responsibility
- Input (gathering, analyzing, and making decisions with information)
- Belief
- Communication
- Learner

The teams I worked on at Yahoo and Google also took these assessments so we could understand our collective and individual strengths and work most effectively on various projects together.

Understanding my strengths has had such a profound impact on me personally and professionally that I completed extensive training and testing and became a Gallup-certified professional strengths and employee well-being coach after starting my company. I integrate this knowledge and training into the health and wellness coaching and consulting work I do with individuals and organizations. It's amazing to see light bulbs go on as my clients come to understand their own strengths and those of their teammates. Personal and team performance on the job, as well as relationships with managers and coworkers, make so much more sense when everyone understands their individual and collective strengths.

I worked with a technology company recently and facilitated a team-building workshop for CliftonStrengths. In this session, we took some time to review each team member's individual strengths. I was also able to build out a team grid to analyze how each person's skill sets could complement one another and to identify where there were overlaps and where there were gaps. The team was also in the midst of transitions, as one person was leaving the team and a new person was joining. The session allowed us to uncover some helpful information that the departing team member could take with them into their next job within the company and the new team member could use to get acclimated to the new team and their new position. Overall, it was a productive and collaborative session. Each team member, including the manager, left feeling engaged, understood, and appreciated for their individual talents, strengths, and skills. They also left with key takeaways and action items to help them progress forward.

Strengths also tie to well-being because when you are able to identify and leverage your strengths, your engagement and happiness can increase, and your stress and burnout can decrease. Understanding and utilizing strengths can also help you become more confident and secure, which can lead to success in many aspects of life. These elements of strengths contribute to becoming a wellness-evolved woman, which is what we are going to continue focusing on in this chapter.

CliftonStrengths, in particular, consists of thirty-four different themes that span across four domains and include executing, influencing, relationship building, and strategic thinking. Executing focuses on taking action and making things happen. Influencing focuses on leading others through speaking up, taking charge, and making sure everyone is heard. Relationship building focuses on building strong interpersonal relationships and connecting members of a team together. Strategic thinking focuses on understanding the big picture and analyzing information to make solid decisions.

In order to feel a sense of self-love and progress through change in a healthy way during different stages of life, it can be helpful to take note of your innate talents, strengths, and skills—the ones that have always been with you from the very beginning. They provide you with the ability to be who you authentically are. Are you more of an analytical person, or a communicator, or someone who is empathetic, or an adaptable person, or someone who is futuristic, etc.? Taking the time to understand these types of innate characteristics about yourself is extremely worthwhile.

Here are five ways you can understand your innate talents, strengths, and skills, which can become a blueprint for success in your personal and professional life.

Look back at your past performance in school, in previous jobs, or in other projects you've worked on: Were there certain subjects you excelled at in school more than others, such as math, science, language arts, or social studies? Did you enjoy certain aspects of previous jobs more or less than others, such as developing financial models in spreadsheets versus building relationships and presenting to clients? If you've done volunteer work, were you more interested in determining the strategy or executing on the plan to reach goals? Answering these types of questions can help you understand what some of your core strengths are based on past work experience and performance.

Consider taking a CliftonStrengths assessment and analyzing the results: If you want a more official way to analyze and understand your strengths, feel free to take the CliftonStrengths assessment (more details at gallup.com). The assessment consists of 177 questions. It's advised that you don't analyze each question too much. Rather, answer each question using your first instinct because that's most likely representative of who you really are and how you would handle various situations. You can take the assessment on your own or you might request to take it through your employer, either individually or with your team at work. Either way, you will receive great insights that you can apply to your personal and professional life.

Check for alignment of your strengths to your current job or career path: Whether you decide to take an official CliftonStrengths assessment or analyze your strengths on your own, it's important to determine if your strengths are aligned with your current job or overall career path. If they're aligned, you will know you're on the right track to set yourself up for success. If you notice a lack of alignment, that could explain a possible feeling of detachment or incompatibility with your job or career path. It could also explain why you may feel stressed, unhappy, or burned out at work. It's important to take note of how you feel within your professional life because it will inevitably impact your personal life as well, if it hasn't already. Since we spend so much of our time working in some capacity or another, it's important to understand the impacts so you can determine what to do next.

Make adjustments if needed and possible within your professional life: If you need to make adjustments in your professional life or have wanted to for a while, take the time to develop a plan. You may be in a position to make immediate changes, or you may need to come up with a longer-term plan. Either way, if you want to experience well-being at work as part of your path to becoming a wellness-evolved woman, you will want to be thoughtful and organized in your approach. Even if a change is required, it could involve talking to your manager about making small tweaks within your current job or assigned projects. Or perhaps it could involve searching for a new role internally within your company. On the other end of the spectrum, you may end up eventually wanting to look for a new job or change careers altogether in the future. These are all hypothetical examples, and ultimately, you will want to decide what direction would be best for you.

Also determine how to leverage your strengths in your personal life and relationships for optimal well-being: In addition to your strengths being tied to your professional life, they can also be applied to your personal life. For example, if you are someone who is skilled at communication, you can bring that skill to your relationships with your spouse or significant other, kids, parents, siblings, friends, and acquaintances. You can leverage your emotional intelligence when it comes to verbal or nonverbal communication to optimize your understanding and connection with your loved ones.

Another example is if you are someone who's a relator, you can use that strength to relate to others in your family and friend circle, which allows others to feel understood and connected to you in a deeper way. When you're able to be your authentic self in your personal life, it can be just as or more satisfying than in your professional life. One of the keys to happiness and success throughout your life is to understand and utilize your strengths in various situations and with various people. It's also important to recognize the strengths and authenticity in others so they can be at their best as well.

DISCOVERING AND LEVERAGING your strengths at an early age, or at any stage in life, can be a powerful part of becoming a wellness-evolved woman. While it's important to acknowledge and work on your weaknesses in order to be well-rounded, focusing on them too much could leave you feeling frustrated and lacking confidence in your abilities. For this reason, I've always been a strong believer in academic and professional settings that encourage you to focus on subjects, fields of study, and careers that bring out the best in you and allow you to be successful and, most importantly, to enjoy what you are doing.

For example, if you want to be a writer because you have strong written communication skills, enjoy expressing your thoughts, and want to positively impact others through stories, innovative ideas, research, and advice, studying communications and working at a publishing company or becoming a professional author, editor, copywriter, screenwriter, songwriter, or marketing communications leader could be a great way to leverage your skills successfully. Or if you want to be an engineer because you're interested in math, science, and technology and enjoy solving problems, studying computer science and working for a technology company as a programmer, web developer, or data science leader could be a solid path to take.

Even if you're far along in your career, it's never too late to go back to school or pursue new or enhanced career opportunities. We will talk more about education in Chapter Eleven.

AT THIS POINT, TAKE SOME TIME to understand yourself and your strengths, how they've impacted you in the past and present, and how you want to continue to leverage them in the future. The self-reflection questions below can help you begin or continue to utilize your innate talents, strengths, and skills in all you do.

SELF-REFLECTION QUESTIONS:

1. What are your innate talents, strengths, and skills?

2. How have they shown up throughout various stages of your life?

3. Do you feel you are currently able to leverage your strengths in your professional life? Why or why not?

4. Do you feel you are currently able to leverage your strengths in your personal life? Why or why not?

5. What can you do to incorporate your strengths into your personal and professional life, and how might doing so positively impact your success and well-being?

CHAPTER 8

HOW YOUR INTERESTS CAN CONNECT YOU TO OTHERS

NOW, MORE THAN EVER, people are craving human connection. After living through the global pandemic, we experienced a few years of isolation away from our family and friends across the world. It's crazy to think that every major establishment where people could connect and gather, such as schools, corporate offices, hotels, restaurants, gyms, hair salons, sports arenas, and retail stores, in every city and in every country, was completely shut down for an extended period of time. It was a predicament none of us had ever experienced in our lifetime, and one I hope we never find ourselves in again.

According to Amy Trafton, in a November 23, 2020, *MIT Magazine* article, MIT neuroscientists found that social isolation can create similar brain activity as seen during hunger cravings.[14] This research shows that social connection is a basic human need, just like food, water, and shelter. Without it, we wouldn't be able to survive.

For younger generations, including kids, teenagers, and young adults, opportunities for social connection were few and far between during and immediately preceding the global pandemic—an important time in their lives when social development skills were still forming. Therefore, it's especially important for these generations to seek out opportunities for connection and continue to develop their socio-emotional skills, which will serve them well throughout their lives.

A great way to connect with others is through similar interests. Whether you are interested in travel, sports, music, technology, reading, writing, history, art, or something else, finding others who share similar interests and passions can help you not only connect with them, but connect or reconnect with yourself as well—especially as you are on the journey to becoming a wellness-evolved woman.

In this chapter, we will discuss ways to discover or rediscover your interests and plug them into your life and relationships. If you are looking to keep your well-being top of mind throughout each stage of life, here are three ways you can first connect with yourself and then with others through interests.

Take note of your past, present, and future interests: Taking the time to understand your interests through different stages of your life can be a great way to connect with yourself and others. Even if your interests evolve over time, that evolution can still be deemed as positive, as you're able to take note of your own growth and development. Old and new interests can ebb and flow, come and go, and come back again, as our lifestyles and the phases of our lives change. For instance, were you interested in certain sports, music groups, or books when you were younger? Did they shift as time passed, or do you still enjoy the same ones because they continue to interest you or provide a sense of nostalgia? Are there new interests that have developed for you during different stages of life? Take the time to be self-aware of your interests over time and see where they take you in the future.

Maintaining your interests or discovering new ones is especially important for your mental and emotional health. Interests can provide a sense of purpose and give you something to focus on outside and inside of work and your day-to-day responsibilities. It's also an act of self-love to discover and pursue interests that light you up. You will have something to look forward to that can keep life fresh and stimulating. In addition, you will feel a sense of productivity. While it's great to have free time and a chance to rest and relax, it's also nice to participate in activities that can generate learning, growth, and a sense of accomplishment in your life.

Determine with whom in your life you can share your interests: As you evaluate and understand your interests over the years, with whom have you been able to share them? Is it your spouse or significant other, kids, extended family members, friends, or others? How do you feel when you participate in certain activities with these important people? Does it strengthen your bonds and relationships? Determine what you can do to keep these interests linked with relationships and create new ones in your life wherever possible, especially if they make you feel genuinely happy. Try to be in the present moment and create memories as often as possible.

Connecting with others through shared interests is associated with longevity. According to an October 11, 2023, article by Dr. Liji Thomas, MD, in *Medical News Today,* people live longer and healthier lives when they have strong social networks.[15] Social networks can bring a sense of support, joy, meaning, positive mental health, understanding, and security and can help improve or prevent loneliness, depression, and anxiety. These are all ingredients for living a long and harmonious life.

Developing connections through shared or new interests in the workplace can also be rewarding in your professional life. Connecting with fellow employees who work on the same team, within the same department, or in the same or cross-functional areas can be a great way to get further engaged within your company. Are there internal trainings you can do together? Are there team events or retreats you can all participate in? Are there workshops or team-building activities you can do inside and outside the office? Find out if these types of opportunities exist, and if not, discuss them with your company and perhaps volunteer to take on a leadership role to create them. Others in your company will likely appreciate your efforts since it may benefit many employees in your organization.

When I work with corporate wellness clients, I often ask poll questions at the beginning of my speaking engagements or have the teams go into breakout sessions while I facilitate workshops on specific employee wellness or engagement topics. One of the key outcomes I noticed was the desire of nearly everyone in these groups to connect with others and feel a sense of camaraderie. I especially noticed this desire during the pandemic, when everyone wanted to feel less isolated and know if others were experiencing the same challenges as they were. When employees share about their families, interests, how they spend their time, and challenges they may be facing, natural and authentic connections can form.

Figure out how to value your loved ones' interests outside of your own: In addition to having shared interests with others, it's quite natural to have different interests as well. It can actually be quite enriching to take an interest in others' interests. It can expand your horizons and open you up to new experiences and possibilities. It's especially nice to keep an open mind and try new things with your spouse or significant other and your kids.

When my husband and I first dated, we took part in activities we each were interested in and connected on many similar interests as well. For example, my husband took yoga, hip hop and salsa dance classes, and attended Broadway shows with me, and I went skiing and snowboarding, road biking, and attended NFL and NBA games with him. Together, we enjoyed training for marathons, half-marathons, 10k and 5k races, weight lifting at the gym, going to live music concerts, watching movies, and trying new restaurants. While life has become busy over the last twenty years with our careers, raising a family, and making time for our individual interests as well, we still try to take part in shared or each other's interests and activities together whenever we can ... especially on date nights!

If you are looking to connect with your spouse or significant other, discovering or rediscovering shared interests or valuing each other's interests is a great place to start. And while it's natural for interests to shift and change for individuals and couples through different stages of life and marriage, the key is to embrace those changes as they come and see where you can adjust or realign your interests. The purpose is to feel connected, which is good for emotional health and well-being.

In addition to romantic relationships, having shared interests or discovering new ones can also connect you to your kids, extended family members, friends, and others in your community. Whether it's volunteering for a specific cause, cheering on your kids at their sporting events, participating in a book club, cooking, hiking, or doing workout classes together, there are so many ways to create meaningful connections with others in your life.

Personally, I didn't know a lot about soccer before I had kids. I now absolutely love the sport, and I love watching my boys play in tournaments and games. My husband and I are their biggest fans and enjoy attending professional soccer games with them as well.

Taking on the interests of others can help you feel even closer and more connected to them. And it's great when they can do the same for you!

IT'S THAT TIME AGAIN to put your learning into practice. Feel free to answer the following reflection questions. This exercise will help you gain more insights into your interests and connections with others as you continue to establish yourself as a wellness-evolved woman.

SELF-REFLECTION QUESTIONS:

1. What are your current interests in your life?

2. What are your past interests, and are they the same or different from your current ones?

3. How do you see your past and current interests impacting your future ones?

4. Who do you connect with in your life, sharing common interests, and whose different interests do you take on in your life, and vice versa?

5. How can you continue to stay connected to your spouse or significant other, kids, others in your extended family, and friends through common or different interests? How can you continue to build your relationships and connections with them?

CHAPTER 9

FINDING MEANING IN YOUR LIFE EXPERIENCES

SO MUCH OF THE WORK I do involves coaching, supporting, and motivating others to live their happiest, healthiest, and most productive lives. And while the quest for happiness, health, and productivity can often be challenging, especially when it comes to making long-term lifestyle behavior changes, the deeper meaning behind what we're doing, why we're doing it, and what we will learn and experience as a result makes the adventure all the more worthwhile.

Most of my clients are focused on goals and outcomes, whether that encompasses preventing or managing a disease state, managing stress, gaining more energy, becoming more active, eating healthier foods, having positive and healthy relationships, or striving to get to the next level at work. While the goals and outcomes are important, the meaning behind them is even more valuable and is ultimately what leads to fulfillment and growth. So, how can you find meaning in your life experiences as you are becoming a wellness-evolved woman, which also involves learning to embrace the changes that come with new life experiences and loving yourself through the process? In this chapter, we will discuss ways to do just that.

Many prominent public figures have a lot of insights and wisdom to share when it comes to finding meaning in their life experiences. Bollywood and Hollywood actress, former Miss World and UNICEF Goodwill Ambassador Priyanka Chopra Jonas is one of them. In an April 23, 2023, article by Jeff Conway in *Forbes*, Priyanka shared her thoughts on her successful acting career and future aspirations, motherhood, marriage, family, and her evolving outlook on life.[16]

Priyanka started out her adult life by winning the Miss World pageant in 2000, at the tender age of eighteen. From there, she began her rise to stardom as a Bollywood actress. After more than ten years in her successful Bollywood movie career, she decided to take on the music industry in the US in 2011, by collaborating with artists such as Pitbull and releasing several hit songs of her own. Next up was Hollywood, where she went on to star in shows like *Quantico* and *Citadel* and movies such as *Baywatch, The Matrix Resurrections,* and *Love Again.* In addition, she became heavily involved in humanitarian efforts as a Goodwill Ambassador for UNICEF. Priyanka also married Nick Jonas, singer and member of the pop band, Jonas Brothers, in 2018, and they had a baby girl in 2021.

Through all of these amazing personal and professional life experiences, she certainly had to put in a lot of hard work and even faced some rejections and hardships throughout the process, including losing her father in 2013. Priyanka found meaning in each and every one of her life experiences. She's grateful for her Indian heritage, her past accomplishments in Bollywood, and her latest endeavors and successes in Hollywood. She wasn't afraid to start over, embrace failure, learn new skills, and take on challenges outside of her comfort zone, as she did when she left her successful Bollywood career and home country in India to take on a new challenge of moving to the US and making it in Hollywood after ten years—especially since most people in the entertainment industry didn't originally know who she was. In addition, after being married, having a baby, and entering her forties, she's found meaning in being more focused on her family and creating work-life balance and stability at this stage in her life.

Throughout my own life, I, too, have had plenty of life experiences that were defining moments in which I found great meaning. Here are some of the biggest ones.

Moving to a new high school district: When I was in middle school, my parents decided to build a new home. The neighborhood was about thirty minutes away from where we were currently living and was in a different school district. So, I had to change schools just as I was entering high school. Admittedly, I was sad I wouldn't be going to high school with my middle school friends, many of whom I'd gone to elementary school with and had known since I was in kindergarten. At fourteen years old, it certainly felt like a massive change, but I tried to stay positive.

When I started school, I was definitely nervous, but I got involved in my classes and extracurricular activities. I joined the tennis team, cheerleading squad, and dance team. I also participated in student council, DECA (a business and entrepreneurship leadership club), Spanish Club, and National Honor Society. And before I knew it, I had made many amazing friends, who I still keep in touch with today. I was also voted by my peers to be on homecoming court my senior year.

By leaning into the new high school experience, staying positive, and getting active and engaged throughout my four years, I was able to take a major change and turn it into a wonderful growth and learning opportunity. I learned how to embrace change, get involved, and make new friends. That was a defining time in my life as a teenager. It made me stronger and more courageous. And in many ways, I'm thankful to my parents for creating this opportunity for growth by moving our family at that time.

In college, changing from premed to business: When I started college, I was on a premed academic track, as I initially had aspirations of becoming a doctor. However, throughout my freshman year, I contemplated if I would be able to handle potentially losing patients as a doctor. In all honesty, I wasn't sure I could do it. I also was very interested in business, especially after being active in DECA in high school.

After careful consideration and thought, conversations with my guidance counselor and my parents, I decided to change academic tracks and applied to the business school during my sophomore year. I was accepted and double-majored in marketing and management. I quickly realized my academic track and major were a great fit for my natural interests and strengths, such as strategic thinking, verbal and written communications, analytical thinking, relationship building, business, entrepreneurship, and creativity. It was definitely the right decision.

And my love for health and wellness, plus my desire to help others, never left me. Later on in my career, I realized I wanted to focus on preventative health and work with clients on lifestyle medicine factors and disease prevention and management. I am doing all of those things in my career now and still utilize my business skills as well. That life experience of changing academic tracks carried a great deal of importance for me personally and professionally. It paved the way for both my academic and career journeys.

Doing my college summer internship out of state: The summer after my junior year of college, I was accepted into an internship program through the American Association of Advertising Agencies. All students in this program were assigned to a summer internship with an advertising agency somewhere in the country. When I received my assignment, I found out I'd be interning with McCann Erickson Worldwide in Troy, Michigan. I'd been living in Madison, Wisconsin, at that time for college, so I'd be moving out of state for the first time that summer. I was also assigned a roommate, who I'd never met—who would also be participating in the same internship program with me.

While I was excited, I was also nervous about living out of state and with a roommate I didn't know previously. In the end, it turned out to be another wonderful learning and growth experience in my life. I became good friends with my roommate, and I learned so much in my internship. The internship provided me with the skills and ability to move around the country for future jobs, graduate school, and family. I also discovered that I loved advertising, which is what led me to pursue a master's degree in it several years later. This is another example of an important life experience that brought meaning to my life and career.

Marrying my husband, becoming a mom, and building our family: Another important set of life experiences that have been the most profound for me involved getting married, having children, and building a family with my husband and two sons. These experiences have forever changed me in the best of ways. I've learned how to love unconditionally and experience love at its highest level. Seeing my husband and sons happy, healthy, and thriving is everything to me because they mean everything to me. I am so grateful to have them in my life, and I want nothing more than to continue to nurture them, care for them, go through life with them, and love them with my whole heart for the rest of my life and beyond.

Losing all four of my grandparents: I had a very special relationship with my grandparents, but for the most part, it was from a distance. Both sets of grandparents lived in India, so I only saw them once or twice a year. Fortunately, those visits were for an extended period of time. When they visited us in the US, they stayed with us for a year or so at a time. And when we visited them in India, it was for several weeks or a few months at a time. I was able to build a solid relationship with them during my childhood, despite living thousands of miles apart and across the world. I also was able to learn how to speak Hindi because neither of my grandmothers spoke English. And when we weren't together physically, we talked on the phone or my parents and grandparents recorded cassette tapes of life updates and sent them back and forth. They all passed away at different times, beginning during my childhood. It was hard losing all four of them, but I am thankful for the times I did have with them and for the unbreakable bond we will always have. I try to keep my memories of them alive in my mind and heart, and I will love and cherish them forever.

Being born with a hearing challenge: This life experience is another important part of who I am, but it is one I haven't shared with many people before now. My family obviously knows, and most of my close friends do, too. However, it's not something I talk about often, and you wouldn't necessarily know about it unless I told you. I was born with 60 percent conductive hearing loss in my right ear caused by an extra bone that blocks sound traveling from my ear canal to my inner ear. When I'm on the phone using my right ear, I may only hear a muffled voice, but I'm usually not able to make out the exact words. So I mainly use my left ear to converse on the phone. And if someone is talking to me in person and standing on my right side further away, as opposed to being right next to me, or if there's a lot of background noise, I also cannot distinguish what is being said.

It can be frustrating at times; however, since I was born this way, I don't know anything different. I've never had any treatment for it, I don't wear a hearing aid, and I've never filed a disability claim. In school, work, and social situations, I make sure to sit in locations where I can hear properly, especially with my left ear. And I sometimes have to ask people to repeat what they've said if I didn't fully hear them the first time. My family and friends often joke with me about my "good ear" and my "bad ear," especially when they're trying to whisper something to me discreetly. Their humor helps me not take my hearing challenge or myself so seriously.

I've had a few CT scans over the years, and my doctor said they could do surgery by making an incision in the bone or using a laser, which could potentially create a new hearing pathway for me. That being said, the procedure has always made me nervous since the work would be done so close to my brain. Also, there's a 1 percent chance I could completely lose my hearing in my right ear.

For these reasons, I've opted not to have the surgery. This condition is something I've lived with every day of my life, and I've come this far, so I feel I can continue to live with it. I am also thankful for the hearing abilities I do have.

This life experience is filled with special meaning for me because even though I was born with this condition and manage it, it has still been a struggle throughout my life. I will forever be humbled by it and grateful for it, as it's made me even more empathetic toward anyone who has hearing issues, is deaf, or has any other disability that can make life challenging.

Now that I've shared some stories with you, I hope you will answer the reflection questions below and dig into your own stories of experiences throughout your life that have given you deeper meaning. There are no right or wrong answers, so feel free to use these questions as prompts and then journal freely and openly. You might find this exercise quite cathartic, and it will help you love and embrace your authentic life and self as a wellness-evolved woman!

SELF-REFLECTION QUESTIONS:

1. What are some life experiences that have served as defining moments in your life?

2. Were you able to assign meaning to them, and if so, what was that meaning?

3. If not, what could that meaning be now?

4. How have these experiences impacted you personally in the present, and how could they impact you in the future?

5. How would you handle these life experiences if they ever came up again in some way, shape, or form, and would the meaning be the same or different from before?

CHAPTER 10

EDUCATION AS YOUR FOUNDATION

"EDUCATION IS THE KEY to unlocking the world, a passport to freedom."[17] This powerful quote by Oprah Winfrey speaks to the importance of leveraging education as your foundation throughout your life. This is another important part of becoming a wellness-evolved woman, as it can help you learn and grow through change across different life stages and also help you find and maintain your sense of self-worth, self-confidence, and self-love.

Education has always been an extremely important part of my upbringing. I am thankful for my education in my formative years, as well as my college and graduate school degrees. Even today, I am still actively involved with both my college and graduate school universities as a student mentor, alumni board member, and alumni council member. In addition, I've continued to pursue training, certifications, and continuing education in health coaching, nutrition, fitness, yoga, mindfulness, behavior change, professional strengths, and employee well-being.

Knowledge is power, and your education is something that is completely yours. No one can ever take that away from you. Your education can also help shape you into the person you are and the person you will become. As a wellness-evolved woman, investing in your education is investing in yourself, which can challenge you mentally, physically, emotionally, and spiritually and also help you see your value.

In addition to pursuing higher education and degrees, there are other ways to learn and grow throughout your life. That education can come through certifications, licenses, workshops, online courses, books, podcasts, technology, work experience, and life experience. Education allows you to better understand yourself, others, and the world around you.

In this chapter, we will discuss the various ways to get an education. We will look at how to prepare your mindset for lifelong learning in ways that work best for you, as you continue on your quest to becoming a wellness-evolved woman who is self-loving, embraces change, takes care of herself, and continues to develop personally and professionally throughout her life.

Higher education: Let's start with higher education for those who have or want to obtain a bachelor's or master's degree and/or a PhD. My hope is that higher education, in all its forms, continues to become more accessible for everyone who wants to attend, regardless of socioeconomic status, age, or life stage. I also hope there continue to be opportunities for financial aid and merit-based scholarships as well. Ultimately, everyone must decide what level of higher education, if any, makes the most sense for them at various stages of their lives.

I've personally always valued higher education for myself and my family. Higher education provides you with a structured format for learning, often with extremely high-caliber professors and teaching assistants. You're able to learn critical thinking skills, collaborate with other students, and improve or enhance your oral and written communication and problem-solving skills. You're also able to think creatively and outside the box, as well as deepen your knowledge in a variety of subjects based on your academic track, major, required and elective courses, and curriculum for each class. Whether you study engineering, computer science, business, medicine, law, psychology, sociology, biology, economics, or another area, you will gain so much from the experience. You will also develop mentally, emotionally, and socially, which will benefit you for the rest of your life.

Certifications: Another great way to build on your education is through certifications in your field of interest. According to an October 3, 2023, *Indeed* article, some of the most popular certifications are in the areas of project management, business analysis, marketing, sales, human resources, accounting (CPA), and finance (CFA).[18] You're able to gain professional skills based on industry standards. Usually, certifications are exam based and require continuing education to stay current. If you're looking for career advancement or to pivot or change careers, certifications can be a great way to help you on your path.

Licenses: If you want to further your education to work in a specific field or geographic location, certain licenses may be required. For example, if you're interested in growing your career and working as a real estate agent, teacher, or counselor, obtaining the appropriate license will be extremely helpful, and may even be required. It's important to think about your past, present, and future career development and what you want to pursue professionally through various chapters in your life. It's always important to do your research in advance and determine which licenses make the most sense for you, so you can invest in the right area.

Workshops: Attending workshops is another great way to learn and expand your knowledge. They are usually instructor-led and can often include breakout sessions as well. Some example topics of workshops for personal and professional development include team building, conflict resolution, time management, ethics and compliance, diversity and inclusion, mindfulness, and mental health. Workshops can be offered both inside and outside the workplace. There's usually a practical component so you can put what you learn into practice. Workshops can be fun and a great way to meet new people with similar interests, professions, and personal aspirations.

Online courses: Taking online courses can be a wonderful and convenient way to continue on your learning path. They've become especially popular since the pandemic, as so much learning had to shift to online. According to a May 24, 2023, article by Ilana Hamilton in *Forbes*, 8.5 million students in the US take online classes at public higher education institutions.[19] Whether you pursue degrees, certifications, licenses, or continuing education credits, online learning is a great option. It can be done in the comfort of your own home or while you are traveling. Most online courses can be taken via your computer, phone, or tablet, making the accessibility factor extremely high. Online courses are great options for both personal and professional development and growth.

Books: One of the most classic forms of learning that will never go out of style is books. Whether you are reading a traditional hardcover book, a paperback, an e-book, or listening to an audiobook, all forms of books provide wonderful ways to seek out and acquire new information, philosophies, data, facts, and stories. According to a December 18, 2023, article by Amy Watson in *Statista*, print books are still the most popular format, with 65 percent of adults having read a print book in the last twelve months.[20] I have always loved reading books, which is one of the reasons I became an author! It's nice to mix up your learning between nonfiction and fiction books, too. While reading for educational purposes is important, reading for enjoyment is equally important. You will still learn new things either way, and your love for reading will increase when you actually enjoy what you're reading.

Podcasts: Podcasts started in the early 2000s and became a modern form of media consumption via audio. Podcasts are similar to radio, but they're digital audio programs that people can subscribe to and listen to on demand. They can be downloaded or streamed through the Internet. You can listen to podcasts on Apple, Google, Spotify, and other services. You can also listen to podcasts through mobile apps and websites and on phones, computers, and tablets.

There are millions of podcasts available around the world that focus on a multitude of topics. Whether related to business, technology, fitness, nutrition, stress management, or relationships, there's something out there for everyone. You are able to listen to engaging interviews that can educate, inspire, and entertain. You can also listen to podcast episodes while walking or running, so you can get some exercise at the same time. This is something I personally *love* to do.

Many podcast hosts also offer a video form of their podcast episodes, which are usually available on YouTube. I've been a frequent guest on podcasts over the years, and I really enjoy my conversations with the hosts and being able to discuss health and wellness topics that can improve the lives of others. I hope you will consider adding podcasts to your continuous learning efforts if you haven't already done so.

Technology: It's incredible to think about how much technology has impacted the way we live, learn, work, and communicate over the last thirty years. Between email, search, social media, and artificial intelligence, it's so much easier to communicate, and information is so much more easily accessible. My husband and I tell our kids all the time how much easier it is to do research and get answers to questions on almost any subject within a matter of seconds, compared to when we were their age and in school. However, it's also important to think critically about the sources of the content you're seeking, researching, and using. In today's technology and media-driven world, there are always risks of fake news, plagiarism, and sources that are not credible. As we continue to learn and gather information online, making sure we are focused on the quality of that information is extremely important.

Work experience: Having solid work experience throughout your career is another great way to establish continuous learning and growth. We learn so much by doing and gaining practical experience. Whether you work as an entrepreneur, in corporate America, in health care, in a law firm, for a nonprofit, or another type of organization, the work you do, day in and day out, serves as one of your greatest teachers. So, take pride in your work and look at it not only as a job, a paycheck, or a stepping stone in your career, but a wonderful chance to grow your knowledge, skills, and perspective. When you approach your work in that way, it will be that much more fulfilling, and hopefully, you will also feel grateful for your employer or business and career overall.

Life experience: Last but not least, there is life. Life is a playground for continuous learning and growth, even when we don't realize it. Our experiences, big and small, teach us something every single day. Whether it's through our interactions with others, being outside in nature, attending various events, going on vacations, going to school, working, and consuming media, opportunities to learn are all around us in abundance. Even the hardships we go through are educational opportunities. Sometimes we don't understand the learning lessons while they're happening to us in real time, but we may come to understand in retrospect.

One of the best things we can do in life, especially in tough situations, is to ask ourselves, "What lesson is the situation trying to teach us?" How can we take the experience, analyze what happened, and determine what we can do differently next time? Being inquisitive and intentional with how we handle situations and learn from them can be a great character-building opportunity as well.

In this chapter, I've provided opportunities to consider the importance of your education and the many ways you can pursue lifelong learning. We are most alive and likely to thrive as wellness-evolved women when we are constantly learning, growing, developing, and investing in ourselves. It's good for our mental, physical, emotional, and spiritual health. We can also learn from others and share our learnings with others, either formally or informally, which can also have a positive impact. Being able to pass on our wisdom from our own experiences is one of the greatest gifts we can give and others can receive. For all these reasons, education is an important aspect of being a wellness-evolved woman throughout your life. I wish you lifelong learning and personal and professional growth.

TAKE SOME TIME NOW TO ANSWER the following self-reflection questions to put the learnings from this latest chapter into practice. Hopefully, your answers to these questions will unlock new ways to increase your knowledge in the future as well.

SELF-REFLECTION QUESTIONS:

1. What types of formal or higher education have you had in your life so far, and have those learning experiences contributed to your sense of self-worth, self-confidence, and self-love?

2. Have you pursued any other types of education in the form of certifications or licenses, and how have they served you personally and professionally?

3. Do you plan to go back to school for any other forms of higher education? Why or why not?

4. What other types of learning do you enjoy—workshops, online courses, books, technology, or something else?

5. What are some of the most important learnings that have come from your work and life experiences?

CHAPTER 11

CORE VALUES TO GUIDE YOU THROUGH THE JOURNEY OF LIFE

IN THE VERY BEGINNING OF THIS BOOK, I shared with you that I had written a personal vision and mission statement for my life. The statement included my core values, which have stayed with me throughout my life. In this chapter, I want to encourage you to think deeply about your own core values and how they can help you live your life as a wellness-evolved woman who courageously embraces change, prioritizes her health and well-being, and practices self-love.

Our core values are often formulated through the teachings we have received from our parents, grandparents, siblings, educators, coaches, counselors, mentors, managers, friends, and other important people in our lives. Their teachings, philosophies, words of wisdom, and other influences can leave a lasting impact on us. Our core values can also be formulated from our life experiences, successes, failures, struggles, and victories. Having a strong sense of our values can help us navigate the complexities of life, choose a life partner, raise children, make career decisions, and much more.

In the November 27, 2018, *Psychology Today* article by Meg Selig, research shows your core values can have an important influence on your health, relationships, and career.[21] This is the last major building block of becoming a wellness-evolved woman, before we talk about discovering your own mission. So, let's stay on the journey together, as the finish line is near!

Through my research and quest to formulate my own core values over the years, here are ten of the most common core values that many of us, including myself, hold near and dear to our hearts, as they can make up much of our moral compass. These values can guide us in various life situations and are powerful tools we can come back to time and time again. While these are some of the most common, each of us has our own mix of values that are unique to us and often define who we are as individuals. What you will discover below is meant as a starting point for you to reflect on what is most important to you and to consider whether these core values are essential in your life.

Health: It's probably no surprise that I've listed health first as a common core value many of us have—especially as we become wellness-evolved women! Valuing our physical, mental, emotional, and spiritual health is critical to our well-being. When these aspects of our health are intact, we are able to take on whatever comes our way in life. We will have more energy, stamina, and hopefully, longevity as well.

Integrity: Having integrity in all we do allows us to make morally sound decisions throughout our life. Life can be complex, and there can often be gray areas in situations. However, if we strive to do the right thing, are honest, transparent, and abide by the law, we will be able to stay on the right path. We will also build trust and strengthen our relationships with others and ourselves.

Respect: Respect is another important core value. Having respect for others and ourselves is essential to living life as wellness-evolved women. Treating others well, and in ways that we would also want to be treated, creates healthy families, communities, workplaces, schools, sports teams, etc. We have the ability to allow others to feel seen and heard, which opens the door for others to do the same for us, creating a positive feedback loop.

Responsibility: Being responsible is a core value that's important for living a successful life. We are able to contribute by helping others. We also hold ourselves accountable for getting things done, keeping our promises, and course correcting if we make mistakes. Being responsible allows us to build credibility with others in our personal and professional lives. Whether it's with our spouse, significant other, kids, extended family, friends, colleagues, neighbors, or others, being responsible with our words and actions can allow others to feel they can depend on us.

Empathy: In our complex world and society, empathy for others is another extremely important core value. It's important to put ourselves in the shoes of others so we can better understand what they may be going through. Being compassionate about the challenges others may be facing may help them to feel cared for and not alone. When we are facing challenges ourselves, it helps when others can be empathetic toward us as well. Having sensitivity for others in our personal and professional lives can help make our relationships stronger and deeper.

Equality: Most of us also value equality. Treating humans equally and fairly can go a long way in creating peace, harmony, and respect for all. Whether in the workplace, in the home, in school, in our communities, or in society in general, for over a half-century, people have passionately advocated for equality in the US. Much work still needs to be done in this area across the world, but since so many of us hold this value, there is reason for hope.

Teamwork: Another important core value is teamwork. When we are able to collaborate, communicate, and develop successful outcomes with others effectively, we are in a position to create win-win situations. Being involved in youth sports teaches teamwork as well. In order to perform well as a team in games and tournaments, everyone needs to put in the hard work and contribute to the shared end goal or objective. Teamwork can then become a lifelong value that continues into adulthood.

Humility: Humility is a core value that involves being humble and having strong character. Being self-aware and able to recognize our own gifts, strengths, and talents, as well as our imperfections and shortcomings, can help us to be well-rounded and appreciated by others. We all have strengths and weaknesses, and it's important to be honest about both our abilities and limitations.

Hard work: Another important value is good, old-fashioned hard work. Nothing comes easy in life, and the more we are willing to put in the work for anything we're trying to accomplish, the better our chances will be of getting the outcome we desire. Anything worth having requires hard work on a consistent basis, which can lead to success and inner satisfaction.

Kindness: Practicing kindness makes the world a better place, which is why kindness is another common core value for many of us. When we can be caring, considerate, and kind to ourselves, we have the capacity to be kind to other people, giving them the space to do the same for others. This is especially the case with our children. The more we can teach being kind to ourselves and others, the better the chances of them being kind to themselves and others when they become adults. It has a wonderful ripple effect. So, the more we all do our part to be kind humans, the better off we will all be throughout the world.

By living according to these core values or considering others that may be essential for you, you will be able to see a positive influence on your health, relationships, and career. Below are some of the ways these influences show up.

Positive influences on health: Being true to our core values is good for our health. When we value health and responsibility, we are more likely to take part in healthy eating, daily movement, adequate sleep, and mindfulness practices. Additionally, when we are living in alignment with our overall core values, we are less stressed. Instead of feeling anxious if we're not in alignment, we feel calm and at peace because we're making choices that are good for our overall well-being and the well-being of others. In addition, when we prioritize our core values, we are more likely to choose healthy behaviors and not engage in unhealthy ones in the first place.

Positive influences on relationships: Living according to our core values also promotes positive relationships with others. When we value integrity, we focus on being open and honest with others. When we value respect, we behave toward others with thoughtfulness and attentiveness. When we value empathy, we see situations through the eyes of others and can show compassion for their points of view and experiences. The more we can put our core values into practice in everyday life and with others, our personal and professional relationships will flourish.

Positive influences on careers: Many core values can have a positive impact on our careers as well. Having values, such as teamwork, allows us to focus on the best interests of our team instead of solely focusing on our own interests. Valuing humility allows us to admit when we make mistakes and stay grounded despite our successes so we can be approachable and relatable to others. And, of course, when we have hard work as a core value, we can't help but create positive outcomes because our efforts will lead us to success.

When we live according to our core values, we have a positive sense of purpose, self-worth, and self-esteem. Life takes on a special meaning when we are making decisions and taking actions toward a path that's important to us. That kind of internal and external alignment is powerful and can make a huge difference in the quality of our lives. That alignment can also be critical in helping us make decisions during challenging times. Core values serve a purpose, not only when things are going well, but when things are not going well and we are struggling to determine the best next step. It's also meaningful when our core values allow us to help others and make a positive impact.

LET'S TAKE SOME TIME TO ANSWER the following self-reflection questions below. By now, you've probably figured out how much I value putting our learnings into practice. It's the best way to embody those learnings and make them a reality in our lives.

SELF-REFLECTION QUESTIONS:

1. What are your core values and why?

2. Have your core values been consistent throughout your life or have they changed in any way?

3. How have your core values influenced your health and well-being?

4. How have your core values influenced your relationships?

5. How have your core values influenced your career?

CHAPTER 12

REFLECTING ON MY PERSONAL MISSION STATEMENT DECADES AFTER I WROTE IT

AS MENTIONED IN THE INTRODUCTORY CHAPTER, I wrote a personal vision and mission statement many years ago—when I was nineteen years old and in college. I have always been an old soul, so that long-ago assignment was fitting for me. Growing up, my parents and grandparents often shared their life lessons and wisdom with me, which I took to heart, even as a child. I have also always had a natural love for reading self-development books focused on reflection and personal growth, which probably explains why I now write books in this same genre to help others.

While it can be easy to get lost through various stages of life, as we all have, having a mission statement as a compass to remind us of who we are and what we ultimately want to get out of life can make the journey much more meaningful and worthwhile. This definitely has proven to be true for me. So, without further ado, it's time for me to share my mission statement with you!

My mission in life is to experience genuine happiness. I want to experience this through the people I'll cross paths with in this lifetime, as well as the things I'll learn from them, give to them, receive from them, and experience with them. I'd like to honestly look into my own heart and know that I've used it, thought and made decisions with it, given it to others, and followed it to the best of my ability. I want to be completely secure with my relationship with God and my spiritual being. I want to understand, respect, and love my true self without any doubts or underestimation.

I'd like to achieve my goals and make my dreams come true, but still live and learn along the way. I want to be able to appreciate mistakes, criticisms, and misfortunes as 'life's little gifts' to help me become stronger and give me new insights and opportunities. I'd like to be able to comfortably live with uncertainty to fully experience the adventure of possibility, hope, and opportunity. I want to be open to new people, ideas, and experiences. I want to find my 'special talent' and my purpose on this earth and serve humanity to the best of my ability.

I'd like to give, receive, and experience love at its highest level. I'd like to have the capability to live each
present moment fully, while anticipating and creating
the future. I want to always remember and learn from
the past, but not live in it. I want to fully discover the
beauty of life and nature and help others discover this
beauty. This is a journey I'm so excited to be a part of
... and I'll travel along it using my heart, mind, body,
and soul!

My mission statement has served me well throughout
my life. I refer to it often—several times a year, if not more
frequently. This tool has been profound for me because it
takes me back to the core of who I am and have always been
and reminds me of what life is all about, especially during
challenging times or times when I've felt lost. It brings out
some of my deepest emotions each time I read it because it's
my true north and continues to be one of my most treasured
possessions. It's a reminder of my authenticity and evolution
as a woman, as well as a testament to my focus on self-love
and unconditional love of others, which speaks to my desire
to experience love at its highest level.

It's possible to have our mission statement evolve along
with us. As I've read my mission statement at various times
in my life, including while I wrote this book, it's been interesting for me to see my own personal evolution through the
years. When I first wrote my mission statement, I was still a
teenager and highly idealistic. Although I am still idealistic at

heart, after experiencing a few decades of life, I believe I am also more realistic now. I have more wisdom from actual life experiences rather than anticipated life experiences.

For example, I wrote in my mission statement about wanting to "experience genuine happiness." My nineteen-year-old self was still learning about and exploring the concept of happiness, and at that time, I assumed it was a destination to reach in life. While I've certainly had ups and downs over the years, I can honestly say I am genuinely happy overall in my life today. What I've learned is that happiness isn't a destination or a singular goal to reach. It's an ongoing journey that ebbs and flows through different phases of life and a feeling we carry inside. I've also learned we can't expect a person, place, or thing to make us happy. Oftentimes, we think our significant other can make us happy, or once we have kids we will be happy, or getting that perfect job will make us happy, or we will be happy if we lose weight or get down to a specific size. Being happy must come from within and often takes effort and the right mindset, which again, is another life lesson that might take experience and years to understand.

In addition to my own life, I've worked with clients who have gone through difficult periods in their lives, which have tested their level of happiness as well. Whether they were fighting an illness, dealing with the death of a loved one, changing careers, or being sleep-deprived as a new mom, which are all challenges I've faced as well, feelings of happiness weren't always on the menu each and every day. That's normal and completely okay. Life isn't about perfection, and simply being human will throw lots of curveballs our way. The key is to tune in to how we are feeling and remind ourselves that if we are feeling grief, fear, sadness, despair, or any other painful emotions, as I and my clients have through many of the above challenges, those feelings will eventually pass, and more positive and joyful feelings will come back again. Having trust, faith, and hope in its return is important and allows us to overcome difficult situations and strive for happiness as often as possible throughout our lives.

When I wrote, "I want to understand, respect, and love my true self without any doubts or underestimation," it was a great goal to strive for, especially when it comes to self-love. However, I am human, and I've definitely had periods of self-doubt and a lack of self-love in my life—when I was in school, during my career, dating before meeting my husband, becoming a mom, and even starting my own business. I was afraid of making mistakes and letting people down, and I tried hard to be perfect to feel worthy of love from others and myself. Instead of trusting myself and going through some of these earlier life stages with confidence, I underestimated what I was capable of due to my own insecurities.

For example, when my first son was born, I was focused on being able to breastfeed exclusively for the first year. Based on talking to my OBGYN, taking birthing classes at the hospital, and all the books and literature I had read before he was born, I learned that it was imperative for your baby's health, immune system, weight, and connection with you as a mom to breastfeed. While breastfeeding does provide these wonderful health benefits, not everyone is interested in doing it or is able to produce enough milk to breastfeed exclusively, especially for an entire year.

The latter was the case for me. In an effort to increase my milk supply, I met with a lactation consultant, pumped and nursed around the clock, focused on my nutrition, and tried to get as much sleep as possible in those first few weeks after my son was born. But no matter how hard I tried, and even after often nursing for an hour and a half during each feeding, my body simply wasn't producing enough milk for his needs, and he cried from hunger after each feeding. I checked with my pediatrician to make sure it wasn't gas, colic, or something else, but what we, as a team, concluded was that he was still hungry.

Since he was born with jaundice and needed to gain weight, I ended up supplementing with formula after those first few weeks, while still nursing and pumping first. I cried the first time I gave my son formula, as if I was doing something terribly wrong. But my mom was the voice of reason and told me to nurse and pump as much as my body could produce and then provide formula if he was still hungry and not beat myself up about it.

Thankfully, this strategy worked, and I continued to breastfeed for four months, at which time I started the weaning process before I returned to work. While I didn't reach my goal, causing me to put a lot of pressure on myself, doubting my abilities as a new mom, and feeling a sense of inadequacy, distress, and failure, I finally made peace with my decisions and knew in my heart that I was doing the best I could. As a result, I had a very healthy and happy baby.

By the time my second son was born, I was more empathetic and loving toward myself because I knew my abilities and limitations. I then applied the same breastfeeding strategy and duration for him, and he, too, was a healthy, happy baby. And both of my sons are still healthy, happy, and thriving today!

As my experience reflects, it can take years to get to a place of self-love, and doubts and underestimation are part of the process we often have to go through in different life situations to get there. What's most important is that we never lose sight of our desire for love and acceptance of ourselves. And, at those times when we can't see clearly through the feelings of inadequacy, having trusted family and friends to lean into can help us find our way back to true north.

One sentiment from my mission statement that I feel I have always been in tune with is this one: "I want to find my 'special talent' and my purpose on this earth and serve humanity to the best of my ability." I knew at a very young age that my purpose in life would be to serve, help, and uplift others. I didn't know exactly what that would look like at the time, but my lifelong passion for health and wellness was definitely a clue. I also love to connect with others through various forms of communication, including writing, speaking, teaching, facilitating, and leading. These are also passions in my life and strong vehicles that allow me to reach and help as many people as possible. I am grateful for the opportunity to do this life work. I am delighted that my desire and my intuition informed me I was meant to help others and showed up in my mission statement all those years ago. It brings me immense joy to know that as an adult, I've been carrying out a key part of my mission, which was created by my nineteen-year-old self!

Another reflection from my mission statement is when I wrote, "I'd like to have the capability to live each present moment fully, while anticipating and creating the future. I want to always remember and learn from the past, but not live in it." While these are great goals to strive for, and I am sometimes astonished that my old soul knew the importance of these aspects of life at such a young age, it's admittedly easier said than done.

I am currently being challenged with carrying out this goal in my life. Our two sons are now seventeen and thirteen years old. Our older son is in twelfth grade and a senior in high school, and our younger son is in eighth grade and in his last year of middle school. While I'm trying to enjoy the present, and I love the stages we are in for so many reasons, including getting to experience their unique and amazing personalities, likes, dislikes, interests, and perspectives, I can't help but oscillate between the past and the future.

Our kids are growing up so fast, so I often find myself reminiscing about the past when they were younger or antic-ipating that they will be going off to college over the next few years. I miss the days of rocking them to sleep, jumpy houses, playdates with their friends, climbing walls, superheroes, and Disney Pixar movies. I miss them coming to our room at night if they had a bad dream and calling us Mommy and Daddy (rather than Mom and Dad these days). I miss helping them with school art projects and the days when they believed in

Santa Claus, the Easter Bunny, and the Tooth Fairy. I miss feeling needed more and being able to help them solve their younger day-to-day problems, which now seem so simple compared to the complexities that come with being a teen.

However, in the present, I love seeing what they are learning in middle school and high school and how they problem-solve, and I love being present to cheer them on in their soccer games and tournaments. I love having meaningful, heartfelt, intellectual conversations with them and hearing their viewpoints on the world. I also love hearing about the funny videos they saw on YouTube, what their friends are up to, laughing at their jokes, and having them comfort me on scary roller-coaster rides. It's also crazy and cool that they are both taller than me now and quickly catching up to their dad!

While I know the next phase of college will be here before we know it, I am trying hard to enjoy the precious moments of the present and look to the future with an open mind and heart. Life will inevitably change over the next one to five years, yet I know in my heart that parenting doesn't ever stop, and our capacity to love and embrace every stage our kids go through is limitless.

One final reflection from my mission statement relates to the last line, "This is a journey I'm so excited to be a part of ... and I'll travel along it using my heart, mind, body, and soul!" I have always had positive energy and a zest for life, and I've definitely been upholding my mission of using my heart, mind, body, and soul in my life journey so far. And I will continue to do so for the rest of my life!

MY INTENTION IS THAT MY mission statement and reflections about how it has served me will inspire you to write your own, no matter what age or stage of life you are currently in. You now have the tools you need to consider writing your own mission statement as part of your journey of becoming a wellness-evolved woman. In order to get prepared, I want to encourage you to answer the following questions at the end of this chapter.

SELF-REFLECTION QUESTIONS:

1. How can writing a mission statement benefit you in your life?

2. What do you ultimately want to get out of your life?

3. What matters most to you?

4. How might your mission statement stand the test of time?

5. How might you and your life change over the years from your original mission statement, and how might you adjust it accordingly?

CHAPTER 13

DISCOVERING
YOUR MISSION

WHEN ALL IS SAID AND DONE, what do you want to be remembered for in your life? How do you hope to live your life in the present so you won't have any regrets from the past or fears for the future?

Living life is a lot like writing a book. You have to take it one chapter at a time, learn from your mistakes, course correct where needed, and keep going until you have created a masterpiece you can be proud of. Ultimately, it's up to you to discover your mission and write the story of your life. In this chapter, we will cover this complex, yet powerful topic, as we take our final steps to becoming wellness-evolved women.

I believe there are four main reasons why discovering your mission and writing a personal mission statement can be a helpful tool in life. These reasons speak to how essential it is to know ourselves genuinely. And what better way to do that than writing a mission statement rooted in who we are and how we want to show up in the world!

Helps you tap into your own authenticity: When you take the time to discover what your mission is in life, you are able to tap into your own authenticity. I believe we each have been put on this earth for different reasons, and we each have something special to offer the world. For some people, it's very obvious, and they know what their mission is at an early age. And for others, it can take some time to figure out. Whether you know what your mission is early on or not isn't as important as figuring it out at some point in your life. It's never too late, and sometimes life experiences are what lead us to our mission.

While I knew what my mission was at a young age, it was at a high level. I knew how I wanted to feel and that I wanted to help others and make a strong contribution to the world, but I didn't yet know what the specifics were going to look like. However, I took steps throughout my adult life academically, professionally, and personally to lead me down a path that allowed me to live out my mission in ways that have been meaningful to me.

Allows you to set important goals: While fulfilling your mission is a lifelong endeavor, it allows you to set important goals each step of the way throughout your life. Your bigger mission will need to be broken down into smaller goals, allowing you to take actionable steps on a regular basis to reach those goals. And with each goal you reach, you will be living out your mission or you will be on the path to doing so. It's also good to remember that your mission isn't just an end state that's a one and done. It's actually an ongoing aspiration and provides the inspiration to continue throughout your life. That's definitely how I view my mission. It's something I am constantly reaching for again and again.

Keeps you focused, even amid distractions: So much can happen over the course of a lifetime, and even though you might have the best of intentions, you may get distracted from your goals and fall off track at times. This is completely normal and is part of being human. However, having a mission statement can help you stay focused. For example, if you decide to change careers, or move to a new city, or get involved with a new volunteer organization, or start on a new mindfulness journey, your mission can help you stay focused and determine if these changes are in line with the path you want to take or if they can get you closer to it. You will be able to evaluate at different times and in different situations if you are staying true to your mission. That's a powerful way to live your life with purpose and intention.

It's something you can keep coming back to: Whether you have distractions in your life or just naturally stray from your goals, you can keep coming back to your mission again and again. It's like the house you grew up in. If you're lucky, the house is still in your family and you can keep coming back to visit and feel a sense of safety and security. The same holds true with your mission statement. It's a pillar or foundation in your life that will always be there. That's a compelling reason to write a mission statement in the first place. When life gets hard or complicated, your mission can provide you with clarity and comfort. It's a constant reminder of your authentic self, core values, and goals. And if your mission changes over time, that's okay too. For some people, it will be unwavering, which is how it has been for me. For others, it may evolve and change along with you and your life. Embrace the journey and your mission accordingly.

EVEN AFTER CONSIDERING the main reasons for writing a mission statement, the thought of writing yours may feel overwhelming. However, by breaking down the process, I believe it can be both an enjoyable and satisfying process. Here are four steps to help you write your own mission statement.

Define what matters most to you in life: The first step is defining what truly matters to you in your life. Go back to your core values. They're a great indicator of how you live or want to live your life, how you treat or want to treat others, how you want to be treated, and what you've already accomplished or still want to accomplish. Also, think about how you want to feel and what you want to be known and remembered for. Take some time to journal about this topic and go deep. This is your chance to put it all out there!

Paint a picture of what you ultimately want your life to look like: Now that you've written down what matters most to you in your life, you are ready to paint a picture of what you ultimately want your life to look like. You may already be living out your mission, or you may be quite content with your life, or you may still have yearnings for more. Wherever you are at this present moment, it doesn't hurt to evaluate where you are now and where you want to go from here. You can still dream about what's to come in your future. Are you still looking for your life partner? Or if you have a life partner, do you want to have a family or expand your family? Are you interested in taking that next step in your career? Are there special causes you want to volunteer or advocate for? Do you want to improve your health so you can run a half-marathon? Are there places you want to travel to that are on your bucket list? Do you want to move to your favorite city, maybe even your favorite country? The picture you paint of your life, at whatever stage you're at, is completely up to you. While we can't control everything that happens in life, we can still have a vision of what we are aspiring to achieve.

Determine the key steps and milestones to help you live your ultimate life: Once you've defined what matters to you and you've painted a picture of how you want your life to look in the future, take some time to determine what the key steps and milestones will be to help you live your ultimate life. Do you need to go back to school or take continuing education credits for any career-related aspirations? Do you need to hire a travel agent for any travel-related aspirations? Do you need to hire a realtor for any move-related aspirations? Is there a health goal you need to hit or a clearance from your doctor needed for any physically demanding aspirations? You get the idea. Putting some stakes in the ground for your dreams, goals, and aspirations will increase your chances of creating your ideal mission and making it a reality.

Write your mission statement as a letter to yourself: The final step is to write your mission statement. I suggest that you write it as a letter to yourself. Writing it as a letter can make your writing more personal, intimate, and compelling for you. It can be as short or as long as you like. You will want to strike a balance to ensure it has enough substance but also isn't so long that you won't have time to read it and absorb it regularly. My mission statement is one page long. You can even print it out on special paper and frame it. It is up to you as to how informal or formal you want to make it. Use your creativity and have fun writing your mission statement. And most importantly, make it your own—let it be a reflection of who you are. You can choose to share it with others or keep it sacred for yourself.

GOING THROUGH THE PROCESS of discovering or rediscovering your mission and writing your mission statement can be a fulfilling endeavor for you. It most certainly was for me. The process takes a lot of deep thought and reflection to determine your life's mission. But I can honestly say, having done it myself, and at a young age, I know it was completely worth the effort. It will enrich your life in ways you could have never even imagined.

Once you've written your mission statement, I want to encourage you to refer to it often. It can be a wonderful guidepost for you, as mine was and continues to be for me. I encourage you to leverage your mission statement to help you practice self-love and embrace change during the various stages of your life as a wellness-evolved woman. No matter how challenging life may get, being clear in your mission will give you strength and help you to overcome those challenges.

It will be a constant reminder of your why and all the reasons to push through challenges and come out on the other side.

WE HAVE COME TO OUR LAST SET of self-reflection questions. Since you will be doing a lot of reflecting and writing on the topics presented in this chapter, you can certainly incorporate the self-reflection questions into your process to discover and write your mission statement. Feel free to do what feels most natural and comfortable for you so you can create your amazing mission statement and enjoy it for years to come!

SELF-REFLECTION QUESTIONS:

1. What matters most to you in life, and how do your core values come into play?

2. If you could design your life in any way you want, what kind of a picture would you paint and why?

3. What steps and milestones will you need to take and reach in order to live out your mission?

4. How do you want to write your mission statement so it's personal and unique to you?

5. Once you write your mission statement, how will you feel, and how do you think it will enhance your life?

CONCLUSION

WE HAVE COME TO THE END of our journey together to become a wellness-evolved woman. I feel so incredibly honored to have had the opportunity to share my personal mission statement with you. I also enjoyed being able to reflect on it, years after writing it. Having the opportunity to be authentic and open with you, as I am with others in my life, has been especially important to me. In sharing more of myself, my hope is that it allows you to share more of yourself with others in your life in ways that are comfortable for you.

Two of the core messages throughout this entire book were about practicing self-love and embracing change. These are the cornerstones of being a wellness-evolved woman and living a Passion Fit life throughout each stage. Learning to love ourselves fully, including our strengths and weaknesses, in good times and bad times, through successes and failures, and everything in between, is critical for our health and well-being.

Becoming a wellness-empowered woman was the first step in rooting our lives in holistic wellness for both personal and professional success. It was about realizing how important it is to take care of our physical, mental, emotional, and spiritual health. It was about putting those healthy lifestyle behaviors into practice, including listening to our intuition, eating healthy foods, exercising, practicing mindfulness, managing stress and anxiety, being productive, letting go of perfectionism, embracing failure, and connecting with our communities.

The next step in rooting ourselves in wellness has been to take the journey to becoming a wellness-evolved woman. As we and our lives evolve, our wellness philosophies and practices can evolve along with us. The key is to keep wellness as a constant in our lives—as that is our superpower—by focusing on our mental and emotional health, going deeper into ourselves, and embracing our own authenticity.

So ... where do we go from here? Along with having read *The Wellness-Evolved Woman*, if you haven't read *The Wellness-Empowered Woman*, I highly recommend that you read it now.

After reading *The Wellness-Evolved Woman*, I consider you to be part of the Passion Fit community, and I thank you from the bottom of my heart for becoming part of this ever-widening circle of women. If you would like to learn more about our Passion Fit community, please visit passionfit.com.

Wherever your wellness journey takes you, please know that I'm grateful for you, and I'm always rooting for your health, happiness, and success. I'm sending you much love and best wishes ... from one wellness-evolved woman to another!

ACKNOWLEDGMENTS

Book Team:

Thank you to my wonderfully smart and talented publishing consultant, Kirsten Jensen; editor, Donna Mazzitelli; book designer, Victoria Wolf; proofreader, Jennifer Bisbing; and publishing advisor, Polly Letofsky, for their amazing support, once again, on my second book. Writing this book was more challenging than the first one due to an extremely busy schedule and time constraints, as well as my own fears about being able to match the caliber of the first book the second time around. Their belief in me allowed me to dig deep, overcome my fears, and find my inner confidence again as an author. I'll forever be grateful for all of them, both personally and professionally!

Thank you to my awesome and fun media and book marketing experts, including Vicky Lynch, Michael Locklear, Hedi Olson, Sydney Bennett, Lydia Vargo, and their teams.

They've really come to know the Passion Fit brand, my books, and me so well, given we've been working together for a long time. They've been incredible ongoing partners in bringing out the best in me as an author and entrepreneur and helping me spread my messages to my target readers and audience at scale. I'm so thankful to have all of them on my team!

Thank you to my knowledgeable and hardworking web developers and designers, Vanja Drobina, Deb Wise, and the rest of her team for all of their support on my author site and the Passion Fit online boutique for book merchandise. Their technical expertise is always much appreciated.

Thank you to my creative and visionary photographer, Marcy Browe, for helping me bring to life my vision for the book cover of *The Wellness-Evolved Woman*. She gets me and always seems to have a great feel for what I'm trying to accomplish and put out into the world. And she captures it on film so authentically!

Thank you to my lawyer, Claire Kalia, who has been with Passion Fit, my books, and me since day one. Her expertise in legal matters for entrepreneurs and authors is always so helpful. I can't thank her enough for all of her help and support with all of my legal needs.

Thank you to Trish Collins, my virtual book tour vendor and consultant, for her wonderful support in helping me reach a wider audience and connecting me with knowledgeable and credible book reviewers for both of my books.

Thank you to all of my advanced readers, including Ashley Jacobs, Kelsey Johnston, Camille van den Broeck, Esther Choi, and Kathleen Ferguson, for taking the time to read my book before it was published. They're all incredible women who I currently work with or have worked with in the past, and I have so much trust and respect for each and every one of them. I'm excited for the world to see their feedback on *The Wellness-Evolved Woman*! There will likely be more great individuals working with me as my journey to bring this book out into the world continues. So thank you in advance to anyone else who will be part of my book team in the future!

Professional, Academic, and Charitable Networks:
Thank you to everyone in my professional, academic, and charitable networks and partnerships with whom I've worked previously in my corporate career or with whom I work currently as an entrepreneur. I'm so thankful to have such intelligent, motivated, and impactful people in my professional life. You've all taught me so much, and I'm forever inspired by all of you.

Friends:
I've been blessed with many amazing girlfriends through each stage of my life, and I'm happy to say these are forever friends. Whether they're from elementary, middle, or high school, college, post-college life, graduate school, my professional career, motherhood, my neighborhood, local, school, and sports communities, I'm incredibly grateful to have each and every one of them in my life. They all know who they are, and I thank them and love them with all my heart!

Family:

And finally, thank you from the bottom of my heart and soul, to my incredible family for their endless love and support. I'm so thankful for my loving husband, sons, parents, siblings, in-laws, aunts, uncles, cousins, and late grandparents. Words can't express how much I love each and every one of them. I wouldn't be who I am and where I am today without all of them. They continue to be my rock, my foundation, and my home.

ABOUT THE AUTHOR

REENA VOKOUN, Founder and
CEO of Passion Fit, is a best-selling
and award-winning author, TEDx
speaker, media spokesperson,
and certified health coach, group
fitness professional, yoga, mindfulness, nutrition and behavior
change specialist, and employee
well-being and professional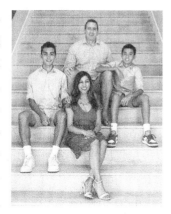
strengths-based coach through the American Council on
Exercise, Athletics, and Fitness Association of America and
Gallup. She is also a personal and professional development
coach and consultant and marketer.

Reena graduated with a BBA in marketing and management from the University of Wisconsin-Madison and an MS
in advertising and communications from Boston University.

She spent years in digital marketing, sales, and business development leadership roles for Google, Yahoo, Reebok, CNET, GE, and Grokker.

Today, she serves companies, nonprofits, universities, schools, and the media through Passion Fit products, services, and content focused on fitness, nutrition, mindfulness, productivity, and work-life balance.

Reena is featured as a TV health contributor on FOX, NBC, ABC, and CBS and is the host of a Women Lead TV show called *Women, Wellness and the Workplace*, sponsored by the Connected Women of Influence. She's been featured in *Health* and *Women's Health* magazines, was an award-winning ESPN National Fitness Championships competitor, was selected as one of *LA Weekly's* Top 10 Health and Fitness Leaders of 2023, and was a Top 10 competitor in the *Ms. Health & Fitness* 2024 competition.

Reena is a brand ambassador for the American Council on Exercise and a Burnalong content provider. She speaks to companies such as Microsoft, Google, and Amazon, writes for *Thrive Global*, *Shape*, and her own blog and has been a newspaper health columnist. Reena has also published her first nonfiction book entitled, *The Wellness-Empowered Woman™*, which is an Amazon Best-Seller, Mom's Choice Award Gold Winner, Nonfiction Authors Association Gold Award Winner, and Book Excellence Award Winner.

Reena is on the Entrepreneurship Advisory Alumni Board for the University of Wisconsin-Madison, Women's Leadership Alumni Council for Boston University, and has been a Women in Management Facilitator for Stanford

University. She was also nominated to be a candidate for Woman of the Year Silicon Valley, where she fundraised for blood cancer research for the Leukemia and Lymphoma Society.

Reena is a wife and mom and lives in San Diego, California, with her husband and two sons.

NOTES

1   Jen Fisher, Paul H. Silverglate, Colleen Bordeaux, and Michael Gilmartin, "As Workforce Wellbeing Dips, Leaders Ask: What Will It Take to Move the Needle?" June 20, 2023, *Deloitte Insights*, https://www2.deloitte.com/xe/en/insights/topics/talent/workplace-well-being-research.html.

2   Danielle Wade and Rachel Ann Tee-Melegrito, "What Are Examples of Self-Care," March 28, 2023, *Medical News Today*, https://www.medicalnewstoday.com/articles/self-care-examples.

3   Ana Sandoiu and Jasmin Collier, "Why Self-Love Is Important and How to Cultivate It," March 23, 2019, *Medical News Today,* https://www.medicalnewstoday.com/articles/321309.

4   Amy Novotney, "The Risks of Social Isolation," May
    2019, *American Psychological Association*, https://
    www.apa.org/monitor/2019/05/ce-corner-isolation.

5   Kevin Leman, PhD and Meri Wallace, "Does Birth Order
    Determine Your Child's Personality?" June 26, 2023,
    Parents Magazine, https://www.parents.com/baby/
    development/social/birth-order-and-personality.

6   Meri Wallace, *Birth Order Blues*, (New York:
    Macmillan, 2014), https://us.macmillan.com/
    books/9781466876286/birthorderblues.

7   Brian Knop and Lydia Anderson, "What Percentage
    of Married Couples Were Born in The Same State,
    Different State, or Another Country?" September 9,
    2020, *United States Census Bureau,* https://www.
    census.gov/library/stories/2020/09/homebodies-more-
    than-a-third-of-married-couples-live-in-state-where-
    both-were-born.html.

8   Jing Luo, Bo Zhang, and Daniel K. Mroczek,
    "How Are Your Personality and Health
    Interconnected Over Time?" June 21, 2022, *Society
    for Personality and Social Psychology,* https://
    spsp.org/news/character-and-context-blog/
    luo-zhang-mroczek-interconnection-personality-health.

9   Hallie Crawford, "10 Online Personality Tests to Take Now," July 30, 2021, *U.S. News & World Report*, https://money.usnews.com/money/blogs/outside-voices-careers/articles/online-personality-tests-to-take-now.

10 "State of the Global Workplace: 2023 Report, "2023, *Gallup Workplace,* https://www.gallup.com/workplace/349484/state-of-the-global-workplace.aspx#ite-506924.

11 "Ways to Improve Social Connectedness," March 30, 2023, *Centers for Disease Control*, https://www.cdc.gov/social-connectedness/improving/index.html.

12 "Learn About the Science and Validity of CliftonStrengths," 2023, *Gallup CliftonStrengths*, https://www.gallup.com/cliftonstrengths/en/253790/science-of-cliftonstrengths.aspx.

13 Jim Asplund, November 5, 2021, "How Your Strengths Set You Apart," *Gallup CliftonStrengths*, https://www.gallup.com/cliftonstrengths/en/356810/strengths-set-apart.aspx.

14 Amy Trafton, November 23, 2020, "A Hunger for Social Contact," *MIT Magazine*, https://news.mit.edu/2020/hunger-social-cravings-neuroscience-1123.

15 Dr. Liji Thomas, MD, October 11, 2023, "Unlocking the
    Secrets of Blue Zones: A Blueprint for Longevity and
    Health, *Medical News Today,* https://www.news-medi-
    cal.net/health/Unlocking-the-Secrets-of-Blue-Zones-A-
    Blueprint-for-Longevity-and-Health.aspx.

16 Jeff Conway, April 23, 2023, "Priyanka Chopra Jonas
    Talks Career Aspirations, Motherhood and New
    'Citadel' Series," *Forbes,* https://www.forbes.com/sites/
    jeffconway/2023/04/28/priyanka-chopra-jonas-talks-ca-
    reer-aspirations-motherhood-and-new-citadel-se-
    ries/?sh=5b753f8b906e.

17 Oprah Winfrey, "Education Is the Key to Unlocking
    the World, a Passport to Freedom," *Goodreads,* https://
    www.goodreads.com/quotes/70547-education-is-the-
    key-to-unlocking-the-world-a-passport.

18 October 3, 2023, "10 In-Demand Career Certifications
    (And How to Achieve Them)," *Indeed,* https://www.
    indeed.com/career-advice/career-development/
    certifications-in-demand.

19 Ilana Hamilton, May 24, 2023, "By the Numbers: The
    Rise of Online Learning in The U.S.," *Forbes,* https://
    www.forbes.com/advisor/education/online-colleges/
    online-learning-stats/.

20 Amy Watson, December 18, 2023, "U.S. Book Market -
    Statistics and Facts," *Statista,* https://www.statista.com/
    topics/1177/book-market/#topicOverview.

21 Meg Selig , November 27, 2018, "9 Surprising Superpowers of Knowing Your Core Values," *Psychology Today*, https://www.psychologytoday.com/us/blog/changepower/201811/9-surprising-superpowers-knowing-your-core-values.

OTHER BOOKS BY
REENA VOKOUN

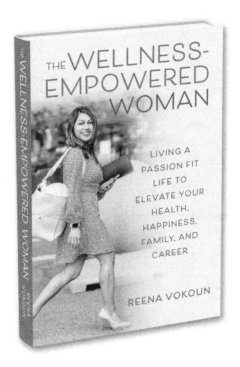

Made in the USA
Monee, IL
07 October 2024

67004725R00100